THE
TYPE 1 DIABETES
Self-Care Manual

AUTHORS
Jamie Wood, MD, and Anne Peters, MD

VOLUME EDITORS
Co-Editors
Anne Peters, MD, and Jamie Wood, MD
Associate Editor
Mary Ziotas Zacharatos, RD, CDE, LD

CONTRIBUTING AUTHORS
Erika Gebel Berg, PhD
Mary Ziotas Zacharatos, RD, CDE, LD
Marie McCarren and Lindsey Wahowiak

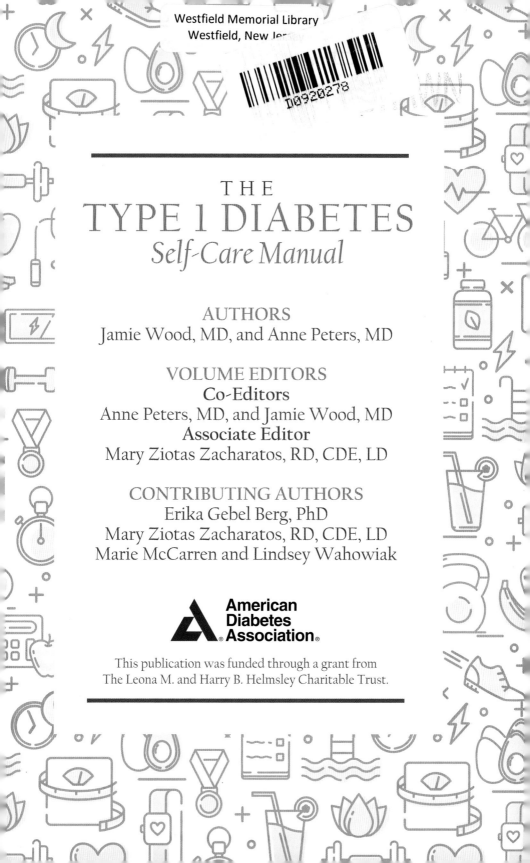

**American
Diabetes
Association**®

This publication was funded through a grant from
The Leona M. and Harry B. Helmsley Charitable Trust.

Associate Publisher, Books, Abe Ogden; *Managing Editor,* Rebekah Renshaw; *Acquisitions Editor,* Victor Van Beuren; *Project Management and Composition,* Cenveo Publisher Services; *Production Manager,* Melissa Sprott; *Cover Design,* Jenn French Designs; *Printer,* Versa Press

Printed in the United States of America
1 3 5 7 9 10 8 6 4 2

The suggestions and information contained in this publication are generally consistent with the *Standards of Medical Care in Diabetes* and other policies of the American Diabetes Association, but they do not represent the policy or position of the Association or any of its boards or committees. Reasonable steps have been taken to ensure the accuracy of the information presented. However, the American Diabetes Association cannot ensure the safety or efficacy of any product or service described in this publication. Individuals are advised to consult a physician or other appropriate health care professional before undertaking any diet or exercise program or taking any medication referred to in this publication. Professionals must use and apply their own professional judgment, experience, and training and should not rely solely on the information contained in this publication before prescribing any diet, exercise, or medication. The American Diabetes Association—its officers, directors, employees, volunteers, and members—assumes no responsibility or liability for personal or other injury, loss, or damage that may result from the suggestions or information in this publication.

The opinions and perspectives of the Testimonial Authors whose content is featured in this work are entirely their own and do not represent the policies or positions of the American Diabetes Association.

⊚ The paper in this publication meets the requirements of the ANSI Standard Z39.48-1992 (permanence of paper).

ADA titles may be purchased for business or promotional use or for special sales. To purchase more than 50 copies of this book at a discount, or for custom editions of this book with your logo, contact the American Diabetes Association at the address below or at booksales@diabetes.org.

American Diabetes Association
2451 Crystal Drive, Suite 900
Arlington, VA 22202

DOI: 10.2337/9781580406208

Library of Congress Cataloging-in-Publication Data
Names: Wood, Jamie (Pediatric endocrinologist), author.
Title: The type 1 diabetes self-care manual : a complete guide to type 1
    diabetes across the lifespan for people with diabetes, parents, and
    caregivers / Jamie Wood and Anne Peters.
Description: Arlington : American Diabetes Association, [2018] | Includes
    index.
Identifiers: LCCN 2017046590 | ISBN 9781580406208 (softcover : alk. paper)
Subjects: LCSH: Diabetes--Popular works--Handbooks, manuals, etc. |
    Diabetes--Treatment--Popular works. | Self-care, Health--Popular works.
Classification: LCC RC660.4 .W65 2018 | DDC 616.4/62--dc23
LC record available at https://lccn.loc.gov/2017046590

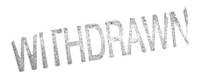

To people with type 1 diabetes, who are simply the most amazing individuals I know, and to diabetes educators everywhere, whom I cannot thank enough for their tireless efforts on behalf of people who need them. —A.P.

To the parents of children living with type 1 diabetes, who are strong and work so hard to keep their children healthy, and to the children and adolescents living with type 1 diabetes, who are the bravest and coolest kids out there. —J.W.

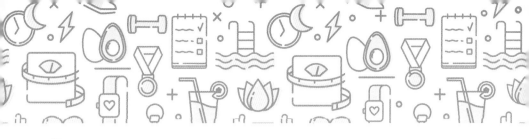

Contents

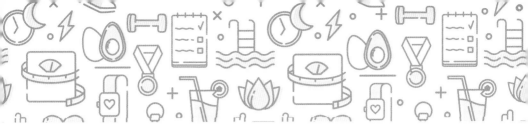

Acknowledgments

This book was funded by a generous grant from The Leona M. and Harry B. Helmsley Charitable Trust.

It would not exist except for the efforts of all of the authors of the *American Diabetes Association/JDRF Type 1 Diabetes Sourcebook* and in particular Drs. Lori Laffel, Jane Chiang, and David Kendall, who were essential to the creation of that book. We are grateful to all.

We are indebted to the contributions of various writers who helped draft versions of this manuscript and patient stories: Erika Gebel Berg, Mary Ziotas Zacharatos, Marie McCarren, and Lindsey Wahowiak.

The ADA publications group has been patient, helpful, and encouraging, and we could not have done this without them.

We thank the members of the diabetes community, our patients, our friends, and most of all our families, who (mostly) forgive us our long working hours and provide an abundance of joy.

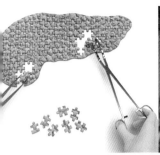
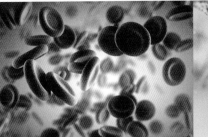
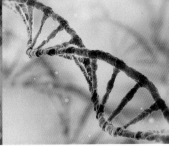

CHAPTER 1

The Basics of Type 1 Diabetes

Diabetes impacts millions of people around the world. Most have type 2 diabetes, but an important minority have type 1 diabetes. Type 1 diabetes has unique features and, contrary to popular belief, is not a disease only of children; it occurs at any age and in people of every race, shape, and size. In fact, there are more adults who have type 1 diabetes than children. This book was written to discuss type 1 diabetes in everyone, from infants to the elderly, from those who are newly diagnosed to those who have had it for many years.

No matter what the age, however, it is important to realize that while diabetes isn't yet a curable disease, it is a very treatable disease, and no matter how frightening and frustrating it is, people with diabetes can live long, healthy, and happy lives. Our goal is to provide you with the tools and resources to help make that happen.

> Type 1 diabetes can be diagnosed at any age and in people of every race, shape, and size.

WHAT IS DIABETES?

All books on diabetes start with a description of diabetes. It is often frustrating for people with type 1 diabetes to be misperceived as someone with type 2 diabetes. Although there are many similarities between type 1 and type 2 diabetes, the cause of each is very different. And generally the treatment is quite different. However, we are discovering more "overlap" between the types, especially for adults who are newly diagnosed, and this can be confusing. This will be discussed in more detail below and in Chapter 2.

> Age alone does not define what type of diabetes you have.

TABLE 1.1   Normal (Nondiabetic) Blood Glucose Levels

Before eating	70–100 mg/dL
Peak after eating	<140 mg/dL

The feature that unites all types of diabetes is too much glucose in the blood. We all need glucose, a type of sugar, to fuel our brain, heart, and muscles. Glucose is found inside cells, where it is changed into energy as needed, as well as in the bloodstream, where it is carried around to all of our organs. Blood glucose either comes from the food we eat or is made by the liver. Our bodies have a wonderful and complicated system for making sure that blood glucose levels are normal day in and day out.

Normal blood glucose levels are usually around 100 mg/dL. Before eating, normal blood glucose levels are 70–100 mg/dL, while after eating the blood glucose levels never go above 140 mg/dL **(Table 1.1)**. If our glucose levels were to fall too low, we would lose the ability to think and function normally. If they were to go too high, it could cause damage to the body that happens over the course of many years.

Patients are diagnosed as having diabetes if their blood glucose is ≥126 mg/dL when fasting, their blood glucose is ≥200 mg/dL and they have symptoms of diabetes, and/or their A1C result is ≥6.5%. An oral glucose tolerance test is rarely used to diagnose people with diabetes, and if the blood glucose level is ≥200 mg/dL 2 h after drinking a sugary sweet drink, the diagnosis of diabetes may be made. In most cases, except in those who are very sick, any test should be repeated to confirm the diagnosis.

Criteria for the Diagnosis of Diabetes

Fasting plasma glucose ≥126 mg/dL. Fasting is defined as no caloric intake for ≥8 h. In the absence of unequivocal hyperglycemia, results should be confirmed by repeat testing.

OR

2-h plasma glucose ≥200 mg/dL during an oral glucose tolerance test.

OR

A1C ≥6.5%

OR

In a patient with classic symptoms of hyperglycemia or hyperglycemic crisis, a random plasma glucose ≥200 mg/dL.

> Normal blood glucose level is usually around 100 mg/dL.

People with diabetes check their blood glucose levels by poking their fingertips or using continuous glucose monitoring (see p. TK) so they know how close their blood glucose levels are to normal. In addition to checking the blood glucose level directly, there is a way to track blood glucose levels over time known as the A1C. An A1C result gives the doctor and patient an idea of a person's average blood glucose levels over the prior three months. It does not replace daily blood glucose monitoring, but in combination with daily readings, an A1C can determine how well the current diabetes treatment plan is working **(Table 1.2)**. A normal A1C level is 4–5.7%. Most people with diabetes should aim for an A1C of <7.5% (in a child) or <7.0% (in an adult who is not pregnant), although patients should have their own goals for what their A1C should be based on their own individual circumstances. For example, a health-care provider might suggest a goal of <6.5% for a person who can reach this without frequent or severe hypoglycemia. A person who is elderly and troubled by hypoglycemia may have a goal of an A1C <8%.

To better understand diabetes, it helps to know how your body uses glucose. Your body breaks down the food you eat into glucose. What's glucose? A form of sugar in the blood. Your bloodstream carries the glucose to cells throughout your body and uses it for energy. To help glucose get into your cells, β-cells in your pancreas make insulin, which attaches to each cell and opens the door for glucose to enter. Once glucose is inside your cells, your body can use it for energy. When your body can't make enough insulin (type 1 diabetes) or when not enough insulin is made AND the body resists the action of the insulin (type 2 diabetes) the levels of glucose in the blood rise.

TABLE 1.2   A1C/Glucose Level Comparison

A1C (%)	Glucose Level (mg/dL)
4	50–80
5	80–120
6	120–150
7	150–180
8	180–205
9	205–245
10	245–280
11	280–310
12	310–345
13	>345

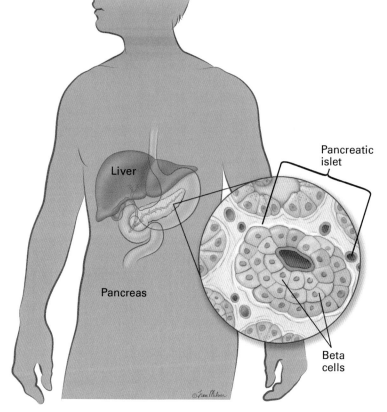

FIGURE 1.1   Location of pancreas with expanded view of pancreatic islet and beta cells.

Insulin is made in the β-cells, which are part of the Islets of Langerhans in the pancreas **(Fig. 1.1)**. These islets also have α-cells, which make glucagon, as well as δ-cells. Normally, glucagon protects us by promoting production of glucose from the liver, helping to prevent a decline of glucose in the blood that otherwise would occur during fasting. But in diabetes, glucagon may fight or resist the action of insulin at inappropriate times, when glucose utilization is required.

In the β-cells, insulin is created first as a big molecule called proinsulin. Proinsulin is broken into two pieces: insulin plus C-peptide. C-peptide is important because it can be used to measure how much insulin a person is making, especially if someone is on insulin shots. We don't think that C-peptide does anything itself, but the more C-peptide a person has, the more insulin they are making.

TYPE 1 DIABETES

Type 1 diabetes begins with the immune system. The immune system has a very tough job—evaluate every cell, protein, and molecule in the body and decide whether it should stay or go. Immune system cells constantly patrol the body for trouble: bacteria, viruses, fungi, and even cancer cells. If these enemies of health are discovered, the immune system mounts an attack. Sometimes, however, the immune system can get it wrong and see danger where there is none. When that happens, an autoimmune disease, such as rheumatoid arthritis, celiac disease, or type 1 diabetes, may be the unfortunate outcome.

> In type 1 diabetes, the immune system mistakenly kills the only insulin-producing cells in the body.

In type 1 diabetes, the immune system mistakenly believes that certain parts of the pancreas—the β-cells—need to be killed. The main job of the β-cells is to sense rising glucose levels in the blood and respond by releasing insulin. In fact, β-cells are the only cells in the body that can make insulin. So, when the immune system attacks the β-cells, it destroys the body's sole insulin factory, leading blood glucose to rise unchecked. And that is type 1 diabetes.

What Does New-Onset Type 1 Diabetes Look Like in an Infant or Child?

The young child who is urinating frequently, drinking large quantities, losing weight, and becoming increasingly tired and ill is the classic picture of a child with new-onset type 1 diabetes. A child who is potty-trained and dry at night who starts having accidents and wetting the bed again could have diabetes. Although it is easy to diagnose diabetes in a child by checking blood glucose levels at the doctor's office or emergency room, sometimes the tricky part is recognizing the symptoms and raising the awareness that young children, including infants, can get type 1 diabetes.

Sometimes children can have diabetic ketoacidosis (DKA) when they are diagnosed with diabetes. DKA is a condition in which high levels of acid, in the form of ketones (substances that are made when the body breaks down fat for energy), build up in the blood because of a lack of insulin in the body. DKA is a medical emergency that usually requires hospitalization and immediate care with insulin and intravenous fluids. These children are immediately started on insulin therapy, which they must remain on for the rest of their lives. They may go through a phase, early in treatment, during which insulin requirements seem to fall, commonly called the "honeymoon phase," but over time, all require appropriate doses of insulin to keep their blood glucose levels in the normal range.

A Math Problem

"Being diagnosed with type 1 diabetes at age 13 was a whirlwind: I remember the symptoms of being tired and thirsty all the time, of going to the doctor and giving a urine sample, of waking up in the ER with two IVs in me, but I can't remember anyone telling me, 'You have type 1 diabetes.' I don't think it happened. And no one ever explained what having type 1 diabetes was: I was told I needed to test my blood sugar and inject insulin before I knew what either of those meant.

Because of this, type 1 diabetes didn't really feel like it was something I had; it was more like a math problem I needed to solve a few times every day than a physical thing happening to my body. To this day, I still find it weird to say, 'I have diabetes,' since I don't feel like I have it. Sure, I feel the symptoms when my blood sugar is out of range, but I don't feel like anything has changed. That's the biggest lesson I've learned about having type 1 diabetes: Yes, you no longer produce insulin, but you haven't changed. You are still you. You'll have your highs and lows (physical and mental), but that's no different than anyone else with or without type 1 diabetes. Type 1 diabetes does not define you."

—Craig Stubing, 29, is a documentary filmmaker and creator of the Beta Cell podcast.

Ten French Fries

"The first doctor was wrong: I didn't have mono, a disease that would last a few weeks. I had type 1 diabetes, a disease that would last my lifetime.

The doctor tried to explain to me how things would work now that I was a type 1 diabetic officially. She said, to an 80-pound 15-year-old, 'Everything will pretty much be the same. Like, you can still eat French fries. You just have to count how many you eat, and you can't eat more than 10 fries, and you have to take medicine via syringe before you eat them.' 'No,' I thought. 'That's not the same.'

I remember the only thing that actually made me feel better. My mom said, 'It's like taking medicine three times a day. You know how Mommy takes thyroid medicine every day.' Very different circumstances, but she tried, and that made me feel better."

—Amirah Meghani, 35, is an attorney and mother of two.

What Does New-Onset Type 1 Diabetes Look Like in an Adult?

When adults are diagnosed with diabetes, they are often told that they have type 2 diabetes at first. This is often due to a lack of an understanding in the medical community that type 1 diabetes can start at any age. It seems more likely that a young adult, someone in their late teens or early 20s, may be diagnosed appropriately with type 1 diabetes, but anyone can be misdiagnosed. Adults with new-onset type 1 diabetes are often not sick at first. Their doctor finds an elevated blood glucose level at a routine visit and starts them on a diet, exercise, and an oral medication. If you or someone you know is diagnosed with type 2 diabetes but isn't responding well to the typical treatments for type 2 diabetes, it may be worth a visit to an endocrinologist to determine what type of diabetes you have. Generally, this requires antibody tests and possibly the measurement of a C-peptide level. The testing suggested is discussed in Chapter 2.

Ten Months of Hell

"I was 50, having presurgery tests, and the surgeon said my blood sugar was way too high. He did the surgery anyway, and then referred me to my primary care physician, who tested my blood sugar again. It was still very high, so he said he could treat me for diabetes. Type 1 never came up in the conversation. He sent me to an endocrinologist in his practice. She was a horrible person and an inadequate endocrinologist. She treated me for type 2 diabetes, with no success. I could barely manage my blood sugars. I'd have to exercise any time I wanted to eat. I'd go over to someone's house for dinner, and I'd have to go on their treadmill before I could even sit down at the table with people. Otherwise, my blood sugar was just going to go shooting up. I hated the endocrinologist anyway because she was so mean.

Finally, I found another endocrinologist recommended by someone, and he also treated me for type 2, with no success. They were all trying different medications, none of which worked. Then I switched to another endocrinologist, who had type 1, and he also treated me for type 2. I tried to persuade each doctor that I wasn't type 2, but they would all say, 'Well, let's just try one more medication.' Finally, I found an endocrinologist who understood that I didn't have type 2.

Meanwhile, 10 months of hell had passed. It was so frustrating. So much of my time and energy was devoted to keeping my blood sugar under control. For that whole year, I never ate dessert once. Anybody who knows me knows that was a horrible sacrifice, because chocolate is one of my favorite foods. Anyway, that endocrinologist started me on insulin, and my life became much easier."

—Cynthia Goldstein, 68, is an administrator at the
Department of Veterans Affairs.

What Is Type 1 Diabetes Like in the Person Who Has Had It for Many Years?

People who have had type 1 diabetes for a long time have learned to live with it in one way or another. Some people who have had diabetes for ≥40 years started out testing their urine for glucose and giving themselves only one or two shots of animal insulin per day. We were not very good at managing it back then. Today, newer insulins and technology can make a world of difference in terms of managing blood glucose levels, but for people used to surviving without these tools, change can be intimidating. Also, many people who have had diabetes for a long time don't like to count their carbohydrates. For many, they have had the disease for so long that they "guesstimate" how many carbs they are eating and adjust their insulin dose by instinct more than numbers. This isn't the wrong thing to do—if it works, why change it? However, it is a good idea to meet with a diabetes educator and/or a registered dietitian every year or two just to stay updated on what is happening in the world of diabetes and to gain new and helpful information. You might want to switch diabetes doctors if things aren't working out, but this might be hard to do given restrictions of insurance plans and geography. Still, seeking a second opinion or finding a way to treat your diabetes better can be worth it if the care you are getting doesn't seem to be working. Sometimes the primary care team is a good place to start when seeking further referral to a new diabetes doctor. Also, diabetes educators usually know who is good.

Through the Years

"I was 15 when I noticed the excessive thirst of the onset, and it took a few days for me to mention it to my parents. I recall being stunned by the news, but I also recall thinking of it as being an obligation for which I would be responsible. At that time, tools and treatment were limited by today's standards. The only insulins available were animal-derived Regular and NPH. Home glucose testing did not exist. Lab testing for A1C was not even proposed until 1976. All we had then was urine test strips. I was fortunate that my father was a physician and a diabetic, and my mother a nurse, so there was a lot of support and understanding.

Age 15–20 (1956–1961): I did the best I could without decent testing equipment or single-use disposable needles and had a fairly 'normal' childhood and college, including hiking, camping, and cave exploring. Diabetes was always there, but I tried to live life as though it were not.

Age 21–27 (1962–1968): This period of my life was spent as a musician, touring the U.S. and Canada. I still relied on my parents for diabetic supplies (insulin and urine test strips) and for glass syringes and needles (which I kept in a small Mason jar filled with alcohol). There were not many hypoglycemic reactions that I recall, probably because my glucose level was much higher than I would tolerate now. This was partially because of my youth, but also there was no method to test for blood sugar levels in the mid-1960s.

Age 28–39 (1969–1980): I finally started to grow up and pay attention to my future, working 'straight' jobs and completing law school. Control was still tenuous (looking back), but I continued to live my life in spite of it.

Age 40+ (post-1981): This era brought major changes to my life with diabetes. First, I realized that I had to be serious about control when I first noticed retinopathy and had a series of successful laser photocoagulation treatments over six years. Second, home glucose monitoring devices became available: first test strips, then meters, and finally continuous glucose monitors that are capable of measuring the rate of change in addition to glucose levels. Third, better injection technology such as a jet injector and fine-gauge disposable needles made traveling and everyday life easier. Fourth, insulins continued (and continue) to improve."

—Adam Cochran, 76, is associate general counsel at a major academic institution and an avid water skier.

All the Things I Teach My Children Because I Have Type 1 Diabetes

1. *It has nothing to do with anything and everything to do with everything.*
2. *It's not an excuse for anything. I can do anything. Except the things I can't do because I'm not 20 anymore. Like a cartwheel. But when I was 31, I did run the Los Angeles marathon. I've had two healthy pregnancies. I love my job. I succeed and fail, and I get overwhelmed just like all women do.*
3. *Having said that, my children know not to distract me in the morning when I take my insulin; otherwise, I might not remember later that I took my insulin, and then I might take it accidentally twice. That was a sucky day, and I couldn't drink enough juice to catch up.*
4. *Quinoa really does taste good with Parmesan on it instead of pasta.*
5. *Thinking cereal is a healthy breakfast is a scam.*
6. *You really do use math when you grow up.*
7. *Exercise really is the best medicine—it treats everything!*
8. *Health insurance is a good perk of employment.*
9. *Be nice to the smart kids at school. They might cure diabetes when they grow up.*
10. *Whatever life throws your way, we can deal with it together.*

—Leslie Kraff, 47, is a physical therapist and mother of two.

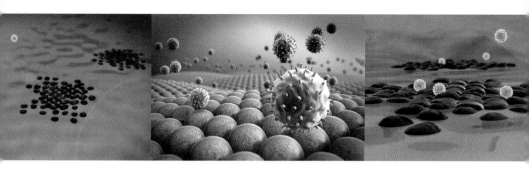

CHAPTER 2

Autoantibodies: How Type 1 Diabetes Begins

Thanks to advancements in diabetes care, such as tight blood glucose management, people with type 1 are living longer than ever. The flip side of that story is that there are now more people with type 1 today than ever before. It's estimated that 5–10% of Americans with diabetes have type 1, which translates into around 1 to 2 million people. While most people with diabetes have type 2, type 1 is the predominant form of the disease in youth. Though there is a rising number of children and adolescents with type 2 diabetes, almost all children aged <10 years with diabetes have type 1, and most teenagers as well. In the U.S., 18,400 children and adolescents are diagnosed with type 1 each year, compared with 5,100 cases of type 2.

Worldwide, 78,000 people are diagnosed with type 1 diabetes each year, though there are huge differences between countries. For example, Finland and Sweden have the highest rates of new cases of type 1 diabetes in the world, while China and Japan have among the lowest **(Fig. 2.1)**. There may be valuable information in those differences. Scientists are studying how genes, lifestyle, diet, and environment—factors that may differ between nations—affect the risk of developing type 1 diabetes.

WHO AND WHY?

While the details remain fuzzy, both nature and nurture have a hand in whether a person develops type 1 diabetes. Type 1 diabetes stems from interactions between genes, the environment (nature), and the immune system.

Family Genes

Long ago, researchers recognized that type 1 diabetes tends to run in families. Overall, ~0.3% of the population has type 1 diabetes. Roughly speaking there is a 4% chance that a child of a woman with type 1 diabetes will get type 1 diabetes and a 6% chance that the child of a man with diabetes will get it. From the positive perspective, ~95% of all children from a person with type 1 diabetes will

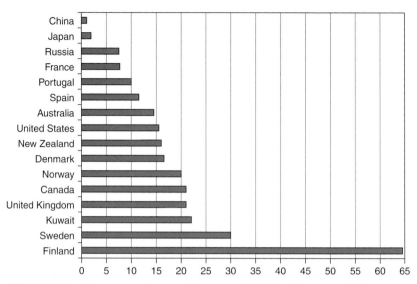

FIGURE 2.1   New cases of type 1 diabetes per 100,000 children aged <20 years per year.

Source: *The American Diabetes Association/JDRF Type 1 Diabetes Sourcebook.* Alexandria, VA, American Diabetes Association, 2013, p. 7.

not get the disease. However, the increased risk of type 1 diabetes in families means genes play a role.

> Approximately 95% of all children from a person with type 1 diabetes will not get the disease.

By comparing the genes of people with type 1 diabetes to those in the general population, researchers have identified a series of genes associated with type 1 diabetes. The strongest genetic influence appears to come from a specific part of chromosome six, known as the human leukocyte antigen (HLA) region. The HLA genes are blueprints for building molecules that decorate the surfaces of cells and help regulate the immune system. That makes sense, as type 1 diabetes involves immune system dysfunction. The roots of that dysfunction may be hidden somewhere in these genes.

But genes don't tell the entire story. While 90% of people with type 1 diabetes have a high-risk version of an HLA gene, so do 20% of Caucasians without diabetes (risk of type 1 varies by ethnicity). Scientists have also identified certain genes that appear to be protective, showing up in only 1% of people with type 1 diabetes and 20% of the general Caucasian population.

Scientists are trying to figure out what these genes mean in terms of how and why type 1 develops, but genetic information can also be used to assess risk of the disease. Several studies are screening newborns for the HLA genes and then tracking those with the genes to figure out why some go on to develop type 1 and why some don't. Other studies include relatives of people with type 1 who may have other genes that increase the risk of type 1 but aren't in the HLA region.

High Energy

"My story starts with the diagnosis of diabetes when I was a toddler in the Caribbean, after an extended period of weight loss and all the other classic signs. The caretakers of the era did not have much or any experience with type 1, so the interpretation of my symptoms took ages. The prescribed care was to apply extended rest and ensure that I ate high-energy foods, such as honey, to put back on the weight and regain energy. Can you imagine the highs that I experienced, along with the resulting lethargy? I was not a healthy kid.

The reverberating diagnosis finally came back from the blood lab—on my brother's birthday. It was not a happy day for me, the little toddler, because the doctors said that I should immediately reverse the high-energy diet. That meant no ice cream or birthday cake. This little guy shed a lot of tears on that day. My good brother was compassionate and made sure that I cut the cake with him.

The mechanism of type 1 diabetes was not understood by my physicians, but my dad became completely engrossed in my care, taking copious notes, reading tons of technical books, and measuring and recording my urine glucose with alkaline copper sulfate reagent tablets.

Many people thought that my life would have been short, but the faith and love of my parents were more than resounding. They took every dollar they had to take me to England for stabilization with recently discovered beef insulin at the King's College Hospital in London, under the guidance of the Harley Street diabetologist Wilfred Oakley, who was a contemporary of Frederick Banting and Charles Best, the discoverers of insulin.

Oakley's words, at the beginning of the 1960s, still resonate in my ears even today: 'Young man, you can be anything you want to be, do anything you want to do, eat anything you want—based upon your carb plan, if you follow your insulin regime—and live to 80, or longer.' Yes, I'm still going strong, without complications."

—Horace Cunningham is a brewmaster and has been
successfully managing his diabetes for 56 years and counting.

Environment: The World around You

While genes can push a person toward or away from the development of type 1 diabetes, genes aren't always destiny. In identical twins, if one twin develops type 1 diabetes the other twin has only a 50% risk of developing the disease as well. A complex interaction between genes and the environment can sway the body one way or another. The three most prominent, but unproven, theories for the environment's role in the development of type 1 diabetes are *1)* infection, *2)* hygiene, and *3)* nutrition.

Infection

Some evidence that infection can promote the development of type 1 diabetes comes from the days before the rubella vaccine. The children of women who had rubella during pregnancy had a very high risk of developing type 1 diabetes. This form of type 1 has pretty much gone extinct with the development of the rubella vaccine, but other viruses may also come into play.

Studies in Finland and Sweden suggested that women who had signs of an enterovirus infection while pregnant had children with an increased risk of developing type 1. Beyond enterovirus, the mumps, measles, chickenpox, and other viruses have also been linked to an increased risk of type 1, but none of these studies proves that a virus causes type 1 diabetes. There may be alternative explanations, however. For example, people with an autoimmune disease may simply be more prone to viral infection.

Hygiene Hypothesis

Too *little* exposure to germs may be a problem. The hygiene hypothesis says that the immune system needs to encounter an array of bacteria, viruses, and other pathogens during early life in order to develop properly. The rise in type 1 diabetes—along with other autoimmune conditions such as asthma and allergies—over recent years coincides with an increase in the use of antibiotics in medicine and in our homes. One interesting observation: an animal model of type 1 diabetes called the NOD mouse is less likely to develop diabetes if it gets a case of pinworms or other infection. The same observation has been made in humans: areas of the world with a high pinworm infection rate have low rates of type 1, whereas areas of the world with low pinworm have high rates of type 1.

Nutrition

Many adults when diagnosed later on in life with type 1 diabetes will blame themselves: "I should have not eaten all those late-night cookies" or "I should have joined the gym with my coworkers." However, the answer is not so simple. Type 1 diabetes is caused by genetics and unknown factors that trigger the onset of the disease.

Breast is best: This research is far from conclusive, but some evidence suggests that a shortened period of breast-feeding and early exposure to cow's milk (before 3–4 months) increases the risk of type 1 diabetes. One potential culprit is a protein found in cow's milk called BSA, which has some structural similarities to a protein found in the vicinity of the β-cells. Just as compelling, though, is evidence that opposes this theory, such as the fact that type 1 diabetes rates continue to rise in countries experiencing a resurgence of breast-feeding. For a variety of reasons, mothers who can should consider breast-feeding their babies, but this should be determined by their own circumstances and the recommendations of their health-care providers.

Cereal and gluten: A couple of recent studies—Diabetes Autoimmunity Study in the Young (DAISY) and the German study of offspring of T1D Parents (BABYDIAB)—suggested that type 1 diabetes risk may be linked to when a baby first eats infant cereal or gluten products. DAISY found that if a baby has their first cereal before 3 months or after 7 months of age, he or she is at greater risk of developing type 1 diabetes later in life. BABYDIAB found increased risk among babies who had gluten before 3 months but not in those who first tasted gluten after 6 months of age. So, these studies don't entirely agree, underlining the need for additional nutritional studies to solidify the links between diet and type 1.

Vitamin D: As discussed earlier in this chapter, different countries have different rates of type 1 diabetes, a distribution that may hold clues as to the basis for type 1. For example, could the lack of winter sunlight in Northern Europe lead to vitamin D deficiencies that increase the risk of type 1? Finland has very low sunlight in the winter, presumably leading to low vitamin D. Vitamin D helps to suppress the immune system, suggesting that low levels might encourage the immune system to go into overdrive and spur type 1 diabetes. However, according to research, giving vitamin D to people in Finland appears to have no effect on type 1 diabetes rates.

NATURAL HISTORY OF DIABETES

Fig. 2.2 shows the natural history of type 1 diabetes.

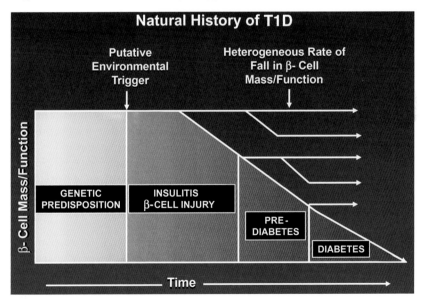

FIGURE 2.2   Natural history of T1D.
Source: *The American Diabetes Association/JDRF Type 1 Diabetes Sourcebook.* Alexandria, VA, American Diabetes Association, 2013, p. 3.

Diabetes before Diagnosis

The biological processes that lead to type 1 diabetes typically begin long before the disease is diagnosed. First, as described previously, there is genetic susceptibility. Then, at some point, environmental factors kick in that initiate the autoimmune process. To get some clues for how, why, and when a person goes from being susceptible to having full-blown type 1, researchers have performed studies in people at a high genetic risk of developing type 1 diabetes to see what changes may take place in their bodies before the disease takes hold. A key discovery was that people can test positive for autoantibodies before the onset of type 1 diabetes.

> People can test positive for autoantibodies before the onset of type 1 diabetes.

Autoantibodies are molecules that recognize a particular part of the body and can recruit the immune system to annihilate that target. In the 1970s, researchers first discovered islet cell autoantibodies in people with type 1 diabetes. Islet cell autoantibodies target islet cells, which include insulin-producing β-cells. Since the discovery of islet cell autoantibodies, scientists have identified several other type 1 diabetes autoantibodies, including those that target insulin, glutamic acid decarboxylase, tyrosine phosphatase, or zinc transporter protein. In a recent study, 98% of people with recently diagnosed type 1 diabetes tested positive for at least one of these autoantibodies. In practice, doctors may use blood tests that spot autoantibodies to help diagnose autoimmune diseases. The antibodies that help diagnose type 1 diabetes are shown in **Table 2.1**.

Studies suggest that people without diabetes who test positive for two or more type 1 diabetes autoantibodies have between a 27% and 80% risk of developing the disease over 5 years. For those with only a single autoantibody, the risk drops to 5%. The exciting part about the discovery that autoantibodies often show up *before* diagnosis is that they can help scientists identify those at highest risk. This group is ideal for studies aimed at preventing or delaying the onset of type 1 diabetes. To learn more about these studies, see the **Appendix**.

Scientists have recently created new stages for having type 1 diabetes. Stage 1 means that autoantibodies are present but blood glucose levels are normal, Stage 2 means that autoantibodies are present but blood glucose levels are not quite normal, and Stage 3 means that the person has blood glucose levels that are elevated into the range of having diabetes.

For people at high risk of developing type 1 diabetes based on genetic and autoantibody testing, there is a third prediction tool: metabolic testing. Doctors can measure blood glucose and insulin levels in response to a glucose challenge administered orally or intravenously. People with diminished insulin production or abnormal glucose levels are at higher risk of type 1. As the autoimmune process continues, the β-cells become increasingly damaged, until insulin production can no longer match insulin needs. Blood glucose creeps up and type 1 diabetes sets in.

TABLE 2.1   Tests to Help Distinguish Type 1 from Type 2 Diabetes

Test	Type 1 diabetes	Type 2 diabetes	Comments
Anti-GAD antibody	Often positive	Usually negative	Can be positive for many years after diagnosis Most common antibody tested
Anti-islet cell antibody	Often positive	Usually negative	Usually only positive within 6 months of diagnosis
IA-2A	Often positive	Usually negative	Usually only positive within 6 months of diagnosis
Anti-insulin antibody	Often positive	Usually negative	Positive in anyone who has been given insulin shots, so only useful if a person has not taken insulin yet
Zinc transporter antibody (ZnT8Ab)	Often positive	Usually negative	Usually only positive within 6 months of diagnosis
C-peptide (should always be measured along with a blood glucose level; may be low if drawn during hypoglycemia in someone with type 2 diabetes)	Early: often still present Later: low levels to none	Can be high, low, or fairly normal	Used to separate type 1 diabetes (people who don't make much insulin) from type 2 diabetes (those who still make some insulin) after someone has had the disease for ≥5 years

Autoantibodies in Children and Adolescents

As discussed in Chapter 1, children are often much sicker than adults when they are diagnosed with type 1 diabetes. Many have had symptoms for about a month. Pediatricians are generally more alert to diagnosing type 1 diabetes (since children are much more likely to have type 1 than type 2 diabetes) and will often order all of the appropriate type 1 diabetes antibody tests. This is usually not a diagnosis that is uncertain. However, in certain adolescents, particularly those who might also be at risk of type 2 diabetes (those who are from ethnic groups at higher risk of type 2 diabetes), it is important not to assume that the diagnosis is either type 1 or type 2 diabetes without appropriate tests.

> There is NOTHING someone did wrong that caused diabetes.

Parents must realize that despite the theories discussed previously we really don't know what triggers type 1 diabetes, so there is NOTHING someone did wrong that caused diabetes. It is human nature to want to understand: "Why my child?" or "Why me?" For now, we just know that there is some genetic risk combined with something in the environment that can trigger type 1 diabetes. Unfortunately, once triggered the body can't recover its β-cells and return to normal. Continued quality research will help us to identify these triggers and perhaps point a way to prevention.

A question that parents with more than one child face is whether to screen other children. There are programs that will do this, in particular a large national study called TrialNet that checks antibodies in family members of people with type 1 diabetes (see **Appendix**). Whether this information would be helpful is a personal decision. In many cases it is a relief to find out that other children are not at risk of type 1 diabetes, but the screening needs to be repeated annually. And if the antibody tests are positive, then research opportunities exist for trying to prevent diabetes from starting. Also, parents can watch out for signs and symptoms of diabetes in a child who has antibodies. But some parents and children would rather not know, because there is still relatively little we can do to stop the disease from starting.

Autoantibodies in Adults

Since many adults develop type 1 diabetes more slowly, over time, and are often misdiagnosed with type 2 diabetes, it is important to discuss this with your doctor if you are worried that the diagnosis is wrong. Signs of this could include being lean, having no family history of type 2 diabetes, or finding that you don't respond normally to typical medications for type 2 diabetes. The most common antibody (and possibly the most useful) antibody is the anti-GAD antibody. If this is positive, you may have adult-onset type 1 diabetes. A C-peptide level can also be tested in someone who has had diabetes for a few years or more. If it is very low when the blood glucose level is above normal, it means the body isn't making much insulin and the person is likely to have type 1 diabetes. Unfortunately, this isn't always so simple. Some people with a positive anti-GAD antibody continue to behave in some sort of "hybrid" form, meaning they do well with a combination of insulin plus type 2 diabetes medications, while others progress to needing full-on insulin therapy.

TIP: Have your health-care provider measure an anti-GAD antibody, fasting C-peptide, and blood glucose level to help see what kind of diabetes you have.

In general, the lower the level of the anti-GAD antibody, the less likely it is to be full insulin-requiring type 1 diabetes. Levels <10 nmol/L and particularly <5 nmol/L are often not helpful in distinguishing type 1 from type 2 diabetes. Finding more than one antibody is helpful, but since most of the antibodies are positive only at the time diabetes starts, they may not be found later in the course of the disease. This is an area that is confusing to scientists and sometimes we can't quite determine which type of diabetes a person has. Thankfully, with diabetes a person's blood glucose level tells us what treatment is needed—if type 2 medications don't work and an increasingly complicated insulin regimen is needed, that person is clinically more like someone with type 1 diabetes. What is required is a health-care professional who will work with you, trying medications and approaches until your targets are reached in the best way possible for you.

OTHER AUTOIMMUNE DISEASES

People with the genetic risk of getting type 1 diabetes are also at risk of developing other autoimmune problems. The ones that are most common are thyroid disease and celiac disease; Addison's disease is rare. All of these autoimmune diseases have an inherited basis and often run in families, with one family member having one disorder (such as thyroid disease alone), another having type 1 diabetes plus thyroid disease, and a third family member having celiac disease. Thus, it is important if anyone in a family has any signs of these issues that they are screened by their health-care provider.

Thyroid Disease

Adults and children should be screened with a measurement of thyroid autoantibodies and thyroid-stimulating hormone (TSH) to assess thyroid function when they are diagnosed with type 1 diabetes. If you have positive antibodies but normal thyroid function, no treatment is needed, but thyroid function tests should be done every 6–12 months to be sure it remains normal. If the thyroid function tests are abnormal, you should be treated so that thyroid hormone levels return to normal.

In Hashimoto's thyroiditis [indicated by the thyroid peroxidase (TPO) antibody], thyroid function is usually too low (hypothyroidism) and rarely too high. The person needs to take one pill each day of thyroid hormone replacement—much easier than taking insulin!

Sometimes the thyroid makes too much thyroid hormone (hyperthyroidism). In this case, the TPO antibodies can be high, but the thyroid-stimulating immunoglobulin or thyrotropin receptor antibodies are also high. This is called Grave's disease, and it should be treated by an endocrinologist. There are several ways to treat Grave's disease, from oral medications to radioactive iodine to surgery. Hyperthyroidism can sometimes be a health emergency. It is hard on the heart and other organs, so it is important that it be treated quickly.

Symptoms

Thyroid hormone is the metabolic engine of a person, and with less thyroid hormone the body burns less energy and everything slows down. People who develop hypothyroidism (low thyroid hormone levels) can become tired, constipated, puffy, cold, or lose their hair (particularly the outer third of the eyebrows). They can gain weight, their skin can become dry, and their body just slows down.

On the other hand, untreated hyperthyroidism speeds up the body. It's like being on too much caffeine. People notice that their heart is beating faster, they feel hot and anxious, their eyes can protrude, and a slight tremor can develop as well as weight loss.

It is best to have just the right amount of thyroid hormone. Over time, too much thyroid hormone can lead to osteoporosis (bone loss) and atrial fibrillation (an abnormal, fast, and irregular heartbeat). Low thyroid hormone levels can lead to weight gain and heart disease. In both cases blood glucose management may be more difficult, but each person differs in terms of their blood glucose response to thyroid hormones.

Thyroid Disease: Child/Adolescent

Thyroid autoimmunity occurs in ≥15% of youth with type 1 diabetes. Youth with type 1 diabetes should be screened for autoimmune thyroid disease when their diabetes is diagnosed and every 1–2 years thereafter.

A child with hypothyroidism may have slow height growth, dental delay, weight gain, difficulty paying attention in school, low energy, constipation, dry skin, dry hair, pale appearance, depressed mood, or feel cold all of the time. Hypothyroidism may delay puberty, affect menstruation, and occasionally cause galactorrhea (milk-like secretions from the breasts).

A child with hyperthyroidism, on the other hand, may feel anxious with tremors of their hands, fast heartbeat, chest pain, accelerated linear growth, weight loss, or feel hot and sweaty all of the time.

Thyroid Disease: Adults

We don't know how many adults with type 1 diabetes also have thyroid disease, but it could be up to 30%, especially in girls and women. Adults should be screened upon diagnosis of type 1 diabetes, and tests of thyroid function should be done every 2 years or so, or if symptoms occur.

A time of particular concern is before, during, and after pregnancy. Women who have positive antibodies may need to take low-dose thyroid hormone prior to conception, particularly if there are issues with fertility. A woman on thyroid hormones during pregnancy will usually need to increase her dose and should be followed throughout her pregnancy to be sure her thyroid hormone levels are in the normal range for pregnancy. After pregnancy the thyroid hormone levels should return to prepregnancy levels.

Some women develop postpartum thyroiditis: after pregnancy thyroid hormone levels go up very high and then come back down, often to below normal levels. If, after pregnancy, a woman loses too much weight, seems even more tired than expected, feels warmer than usual, and has an increase in heart rate, this could be the problem. Thyroid function should be tested. Treatment is often not needed for postpartum high thyroid hormone levels but is needed if low thyroid hormone levels follow.

Celiac Disease

Celiac disease is a common immune disease of the small intestine that occurs in genetically susceptible individuals when they eat gluten (or more specifically the gliadin moiety of gluten), which is found in wheat, rye, barley, and possibly oats. The antibodies damage the lining of the small intestines, which makes it harder for the intestines to absorb food and needed vitamins. People who develop celiac disease often have diarrhea and may have weight loss, bloating, and pain in their abdomen.

Celiac Disease: Child/Adolescent

It seems as though children diagnosed with type 1 diabetes are more likely to develop celiac disease than adults diagnosed with diabetes, but we don't know for sure. In children diagnosed with type 1 diabetes, rates of celiac disease may be up to 10%. Therefore, after the diagnosis of type 1 diabetes and stabilization of blood glucose levels, your child should have a celiac panel: measurements of tissue transglutaminase, anti-endomysial, and/or deamidated gliadin IgA antibodies, with documentation of normal total serum IgA levels. Your child must be eating gluten for these tests to be helpful—avoiding gluten can lower the levels of these antibodies and make the diagnosis difficult.

Symptoms in a child include a falloff in growth rate as well as a loss of weight and BMI percentile. There may be unexplained hypo- or hyperglycemia due to the disordered absorption of food, often leading to suboptimal glycemic control with high glucose variability.

Children with positive antibodies should be referred to a gastroenterologist. The gastroenterologist will consider whether a biopsy of the intestines is required to confirm the diagnosis.

If your child has celiac disease, he or she must follow a gluten-free diet for life so that the intestines work properly and stay healthy. Work closely with a registered dietitian who specializes in both celiac disease and type 1 diabetes nutritional management.

If the initial screen for celiac is negative, the test should be repeated every 2 years or if symptoms of celiac disease develop. We do not know exactly how often to screen children for celiac disease or how long to keep testing. Ask for screening if symptoms are present or it has been ≥2 years since the last test.

Celiac Disease: Adults

Celiac disease can develop during adulthood, but we know less about the need to screen adult patients than we do for children. Certainly adults with symptoms should be screened. These symptoms include diarrhea, bloating, abdominal pain, weight loss, erratic blood glucose levels, osteoporosis, and vitamin D deficiency. In addition, if there is a family history of autoimmune disease, such as celiac or thyroid disease, screening should be done. False negative results are possible if the person has not eaten gluten in a while. As for adult patients with new-onset type 1 diabetes and no symptoms or family history, we do not know if screening is helpful. Additionally, the test may not be covered by all insurance plans in adults who do not have symptoms. Therefore, this is something you should discuss with your doctor.

Addison's Disease (Adrenal Insufficiency)

Very rarely, a person's immune system destroys the adrenal glands. This is very serious because the adrenal glands make cortisol, which is required for life. This condition is called Addison's disease or adrenal insufficiency.

In people with type 1 diabetes, a clue to the presence of Addison's disease is a change in the pattern of low blood glucose levels. Cortisol is one of the hormones that helps keep blood glucose levels normal, and without it blood glucose levels would fall more rapidly and more often. People may start to have very serious low blood glucose reactions and notice that they need a lot less insulin to manage their blood glucose levels.

Other clues include a darkening of the skin, which is often seen if there is a cut that forms a scar or a scar caused by a surgeon. People with Addison's disease also lose weight, feel very tired, crave salt, and may start to feel lightheaded and dizzy when they stand up. They may have nausea, vomiting, and occasional diarrhea.

Screening for Addison's disease is not recommended in adults or children with type 1 diabetes because it is so rare. But if someone with type 1 diabetes develops the signs and symptoms discussed previously they should be checked to see if their body is making enough cortisol. The treatment is to replace cortisol, and it is taken as an oral tablet two to three times per day.

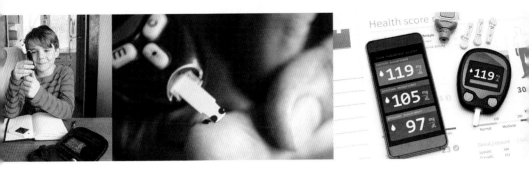

CHAPTER 3

Your Blood Glucose Goals

People are now living long, healthy, and active lives with diabetes. Advances in treatments and technologies have helped cause these improvements, but it is the people with diabetes themselves who have learned how to use these treatments to improve their health. We know what it takes to live long and prosper with type 1.

A LANDMARK STUDY LIVES ON

Insulin, while amazing, unfortunately is not a cure for diabetes. In the decades after insulin's discovery, it became clear that, even with insulin injections, people with diabetes often developed serious complications, such as blindness, amputations, and kidney failure. No one knew why these complications occurred or how to prevent them. The problem was that it wasn't yet clear how best to use insulin. Up until the 1980s, the conventional treatment for type 1 diabetes was a shot or two of insulin a day, and that was that. Convenience was king and technology was lacking.

> The DCCT study had proven that managing diabetes can lead to a healthier life with less risk of developing diabetes-related disease.

Technological advances, such as portable blood glucose meters, insulin pens and pumps, made it possible to step up diabetes management. An approach to diabetes treatment called "intensive therapy" emerged. It required close monitoring of blood glucose levels, multiple daily injections or a pump, and a multidisciplinary team of health-care providers. The idea was to prevent complications by keeping blood glucose levels as close to levels seen in people without diabetes as possible. However, intensive treatment was expensive, difficult, and time-consuming, and there wasn't evidence that it kept people with type 1 diabetes any healthier than conventional care. That is, until the Diabetes Control and Complications Trial (DCCT).

The goal of DCCT was simple: figure out whether keeping blood glucose levels closer to normal could lower the risk of long-term diabetes complications. The study itself, though, was a herculean effort. The study included 1,441 participants and lasted >6 years.

Half the participants followed a conventional approach while the rest were intensively treated. The participants in the intensive group were encouraged to check blood glucose levels four to seven times a day and use the information to make decisions about insulin, food, and activity. The goal was to achieve blood glucose levels close to those of a person not living with diabetes as safely as possible. The intensively treated patients were able to reach an average A1C of 7.2% compared with an A1C of 9% in the control (conventional) group.

The results were so clear, so resounding, that the trial was halted a year early: members of the intensive group had less than half the risk of developing diabetes-related eye, kidney, and nerve disease. DCCT had proven that managing diabetes could lead to a healthier life with less risk of developing a diabetes-related disease.

Each person with type 1 diabetes should have their own personal A1C goal.

YOUR GOALS

Each person with type 1 diabetes should have their own personal A1C goal (**Tables 3.1 and 3.2**). Set your target along with your health-care provider. Your goal will be based on a number of factors. The general A1C target is <7.5% for people aged <18 years and <7% for those aged ≥18 years, but these targets vary a lot depending on the individual. The closer to normal the blood glucose levels are, the less risk of the long-term complications of diabetes. However, this has to be balanced against the risk of low blood glucose reactions.

TABLE 3.1   American Diabetes Association Recommendations for Most Nonpregnant Adults

A1C	<7%*
Before meals	80–130 mg/dL
Peak blood glucose after meals (1–2 h)	<180 mg/dL

*More or less stringent glycemic goals may be appropriate for individual patients. Goals should be individualized based on the duration of diabetes, age/life expectancy, comorbid conditions, known cardiovascular disease or advanced microvascular complications, hypoglycemia unawareness, and individual patient considerations.

TABLE 3.2   American Diabetes Association Guidelines

Age	Health	A1C (%)
Youth (<18 years)	Not pregnant	<7.5
Adults	Not pregnant	<7.0
Older adults (≥65 years)	Healthy; long life expected	<7.5
Older adults	Some health issues	<8.0
Older adults	Poor health	<8.5

> Never let anyone intimidate you or your child by saying, "Your A1C should be x, y, or z."

You are unique and need advice based on your own set of circumstances. Never let anyone intimidate you or your child by saying, "Your A1C level should be x, y, or z." Your response can be: "I am working with my health care provider on reaching my own safe diabetes target, and it has been customized for my own condition."

A1C targets often change over time, sometimes decreasing and sometimes increasing. It all depends on the person. Don't compare yourself or your child to others. You know how hard you are trying and what your goals are. Be clear, persistent, and honest in your approach. Never avoid going to see your health-care team because you feel like a "failure." The members of your medical team are your coaches. They understand that multiple life challenges influence diabetes each day and night. An A1C is what it is; life changes, and you need support all along the way to stay the same or improve. It is all part of the process of living with diabetes.

It's Not a Race

"I can upload the data stored on my pump and read it in chart or graph form to look for particular patterns over a period of time so that I can make corrections in my regimen. When I go to see a physician I have a lot of information with me beforehand. We are both better informed. However, sometimes the data can be overwhelming. There are trade-offs when using the latest devices. If I'm doing well, do I really need to be doing 'better'? It's essential for me to remember that what's important is to live well with diabetes, not to control it. The only reason for 'controlling' (not a term I like) the disease is to continue to live a happy life. Getting everything correct is not a moral issue. It's not a race or a competition. There are so many variables that one can never get it perfect. It's not a battle. It's a way of living. My body doesn't produce insulin and yet here I am, still having fun, and I don't necessarily need to have more and quicker data to do it."

—Drew Wickman, 70, is a teacher and potter who has had
type 1 diabetes since 1948.

SELF-MONITORING OF BLOOD GLUCOSE

One of the first tasks that patients and/or caregivers must learn is how to measure blood glucose levels. This means getting a drop of blood on a strip that is inserted into a meter that measures the blood glucose level or wearing a factory calibrated continuous glucose monitor (see below). For many, checking blood glucose is one of the parts of having type 1 diabetes that is the most difficult. It hurts a little, and some people are self-conscious about doing it in front of other people.

> Knowing how to react to different blood glucose levels is an ongoing task that you/your child will work on with your health-care team.

Once the meter tells you your blood glucose level, you will have to know what to do with the information. Knowing how to react to different blood glucose levels is an ongoing task that you/your child will work on with your health-care team.

Fingerstick Checking

First you must assemble the pieces and learn how to use them **(Fig. 3.1)**. The parts needed include *1)* a lancing device (the plastic stick that holds the lancet and pushes it down into the finger), *2)* lancets (the devices that do the poking), *3)* a test strip, and *4)* a meter (which tells you the blood glucose number).

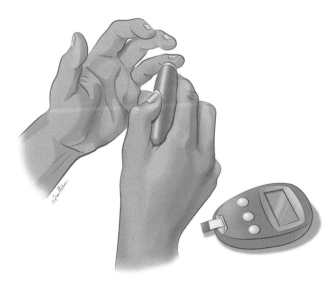

FIGURE 3.1   People with diabetes typically use a lancing device to obtain a blood sample when using a glucose meter to check their blood glucose level in the sample.

Lancing Device

Each brand of meter comes with its own type of lancing device, although they are all pretty similar. They can be set to varying depths. Start at the lowest level for the gentlest poke. Depending on your/your child's skin, you may need a different setting. Find the one that is best. You do not have to use the lancet that comes with the meter you chose. Many people use a meter and lancet from different manufacturers.

Some lancing devices can be used to get a sample of blood from the forearm. Usually this requires using a different cap. Follow the instructions that come with the device. Checking blood from the arm is slightly less accurate and may not be much less painful than the fingertip. If blood glucose levels are changing quickly or you suspect a low level, use fingersticks. Speak to your diabetes team, but in general, checking blood glucose levels on the forearm is discouraged in children.

Lancets

Be sure to ask your health-care provider for the lancet you prefer. Some devices take only one lancet at a time. Others have a little cartridge that holds several lancets, and the device automatically rotates to a new lancet. In practice, people often use the same lancet over and over. The more it is used, the duller it becomes. We recommend changing the lancet at least once a day. If you/your child is very sensitive to fingersticks, it is good to use a new one each time.

Test Strips

Each brand of meter has its own test strips. They are not interchangeable. Test strips must be kept covered in the little bottle they come in or in their foil wrappings. Don't use expired test strips because they may not be accurate. Tell your health-care provider exactly which strips are needed and how often you check your blood glucose.

Meters

There are many meters on the market and some are better than others. Ask your health-care provider which they prefer and which meters your insurance company will cover. Some meters work with specific pumps. Others work with certain Internet applications and programs; others have Bluetooth and other capacities for communicating data, all of which can be helpful for diabetes management. Each meter comes with instructions in the box as well as online.

Some meters are small; some are big. Some come in pretty colors. Some have larger numbers and light up. Some tell you if your blood glucose level is too high or too low. Regardless of the exact type of meter, it should be something you/your child feels comfortable using. Often it helps to have more than one meter set up for easy checking.

> Your health care provider needs to actually look at your blood glucose records at each visit.

Your health-care provider needs to actually look at your blood glucose records at each visit. Bring all the meters and monitors that you/your child uses to your appointments, plus any records of blood glucose levels and any completed food records. Even if it's just a few days' worth, it's helpful for your diabetes health-care team. The only way diabetes can be well managed is with blood glucose checking, and the more that is given to your health-care provider, the better the visit will be. Once a year, *Diabetes Forecast* discusses all the various type of meters and their pros and cons in their annual consumer guide.

Accuracy

People are often frustrated by how much blood glucose levels can vary even if taken just a few minutes apart. It seems as if there is no "truth" as to what the blood glucose level is and this can be very confusing. Trust your instincts. If a result seems wrong, check again. The following are common reasons why blood glucose levels seem to vary:

1. The U.S. Food and Drug Administration (FDA): The standard for approving blood glucose meters means that there is an accepted variance of 10–15% with an occasional level that may be erroneously high. Usually meters are more accurate in the low range.

2. Expired strips: This adds a level of variability and these results should not be trusted.

3. Sugar on fingertips: Touching something that contains sugar—a powdered donut, orange slices—can make the meter reading too high. Even dirt on the fingers can falsely raise the measured glucose level. Before checking a blood glucose level, wash your hands. If a blood glucose level seems far too high, then wash your/your child's hands and check it again. Another trick is to prick the finger, wipe off the first drop of blood with a tissue, and then use the second drop of blood to check the glucose.

4. Too little blood: The blood glucose level can read too low if there is not enough blood on the test strip. This happens rarely, because meters generally won't read the glucose level if not enough blood is present, and the meter will usually show an error message, but it is worth considering.

5. Altitude: Some meters don't work as well at high altitudes. Discuss this with your health-care provider if you are going to spend time at altitudes >10,000 feet. Anecdotally some people find their blood glucose levels read higher, whereas some find their blood glucose meter reads lower. You may want to carry more than one type of meter or raise blood glucose targets during your trip.

6. Wet fingers: Sometimes the blood glucose reading will be falsely low if the fingers were still wet from washing them or using alcohol. The moisture on the finger dilutes the blood drop and lowers the reading. Make sure that fingers are dry before checking a blood glucose.

Use of a Blood Glucose Meter for Self-Management of Diabetes through the Life Span

Infants: It takes infants a few days or weeks to adjust to having their blood glucose levels checked, and they may cry or resist. Be loving and caring, but firm and consistent, that the blood glucose needs to be checked. Allowing your baby to delay the blood glucose check with a tantrum will cause more problems down the road. It helps to have one caregiver hold the child in a warm bear hug, giving encouragement and affection, while another caregiver checks the blood glucose. Some caregivers find checking toes easier, especially at night. This is only recommended in an infant who is not yet walking. Encourage the infant to help with the task; they may be able to hold out their finger or hold the alcohol pad.

Children: Toddlers love to help with the steps; they can help gather the supplies, hold things, and clean their own finger. By the age of 3 years most children have the dexterity to check their own blood glucose, but of course they should always be supervised. Although there is a lot of variability, most school-aged children know if a reading is low, in range, or high but need help to decide what to do next. By middle school, most children can independently check their blood glucose, interpret the value, and know what to do next.

Adults: Removing the lancet from the lancing device can be difficult for older people, especially those with limited dexterity. To obtain a drop of blood, it's helpful to wash the hands in warm water and dangle the arm below the heart to use gravity to create the drop. Over time, you will develop some calluses on your favorite fingertips, so you may need to increase the depth of the fingerstick on the lancet. Rotate the sites you use.

How Often and When to Check

More frequent checking is associated with a lower A1C. Your health-care team will help you decide how often to check. For starters it's good to check before each meal and at bedtime (four times a day). You may need to check between meals, if you feel low, and before exercise or driving. Some people need to check ≥10 times a day to achieve their goals. However, if you have a continuous glucose monitor (see next section) you may not have to do fingersticks or only need to do so to calibrate **(Fig. 3.2)**.

It's a Marathon, Not a Sprint

"Take a long view of things. It's a marathon, not a sprint. Do your best today. If it's not good, then tomorrow can be. No one goes days without a couple of unusually high readings. Sometimes they make you feel incompetent—can't tell you how many times in a doctor's office they will say something like, 'Is your blood sugar ever over 200?' Of course it is! The point is to try your best every day. You're playing a long game."

—Jim Urie, 64, a retired music company executive, has had
type 1 diabetes since 1968.

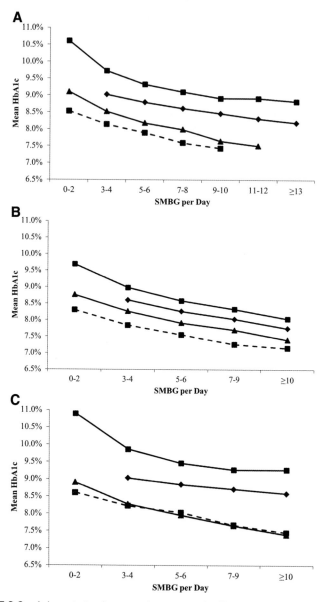

FIGURE 3.2   *A:* Association between frequency of self-monitoring of blood glucose per day and A1C. *B:* Pump users only. *C:* Injection users only. Solid black line and diamonds: age 1 year to younger than 13. Solid black line and squares: age 13 years to younger than 26. Solid black line and triangle: age 26 years to younger than 50. Dotted black line and squares: age 50 years and older.

Source: Miller, Evidence of a strong association between frequency of self-monitoring of blood glucose and hemoglobin A1c levels in T1D exchange clinic registry participants. *Diabetes Care* 2013;36:2009–2014.

Like a Tennis Match

"Today, self-management is much easier than when I got type 1 in 1969. Looking at test tape for rough approximations of glucose presence in my urine was like looking at a star in the sky: I could see something, but I did not know much about it. Now my glucose levels are graphed for me, available in a couple of seconds, and retrievable on a small receiver in my pocket or on my phone. I don't have to guess what direction my glucose is headed. It's like a tennis match, but you know where your opponent will hit the next shot and how hard it will be hit. I like those odds."

— Peter Madden, 60, is an accountant working in aerospace.

Continuous Glucose Monitoring

Continuous glucose monitoring (CGM) is a tool that that has changed how diabetes is managed for people with type 1 diabetes **(Fig. 3.3)**.

Whether you/your child uses shots or a pump, you can use a CGM system. A small sensor is inserted under the skin and sends a signal via a transmitter to a receiver (either a separate receiver or a smartphone or an insulin pump). It tells you what the glucose level is every few minutes and gives trends to indicate if blood glucose levels are falling, rising, or staying the same. Sensors can be worn in the same areas in which injections are given. Many people wear them in their abdominal area or on the back of the arm.

These systems have three pieces: the sensor, the transmitter, and the receiver.

The part of the sensor that goes under the skin is tiny, like a 1-cm piece of fishing line. An inserter device with a metal guide pushes the sensor under the skin and then is withdrawn. This process is relatively painless, although one can feel the sensor going under the skin. The sensor needs to be changed every week or so. Most need to be calibrated against a fingerstick blood glucose level 2–4 times a day.

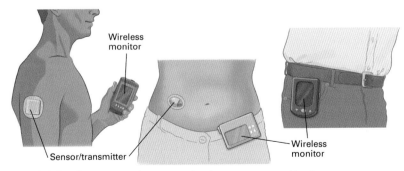

FIGURE 3.3   Continuous glucose monitoring systems provide glucose measurements as often as once per minute. The measurements are transmitted to a wireless monitor.

Described below is the use of rtCGM (real time CGM). The Abbott Libre is a different form of CGM—it does not require calibration, but does not give alerts and alarms for rising or falling blood glucose levels. It can be very helpful to obtain a blood glucose value with trend arrows.

The sensor reads the fluid in the tissue just below the skin, known as the interstitial fluid, so that there may be a difference between the level measured by a blood fingerstick and by the sensor, especially when the glucose in the blood is rising or falling quickly. Sensors are helpful for trends because they indicate whether the blood glucose level is going up or down. For the sensor (which works with the Medtronic pump), it is recommended that users confirm values with their meter before giving insulin or treating a low glucose level. The Dexcom G5 has been approved as a strip replacement by the FDA, which means users can dose off the numbers provided by the sensor. However, the sensor needs to be calibrated twice a day with fingersticks. Of course, if there is any concern as to the accuracy of the sensor reading, a fingerstick should be done to confirm the glucose reading, especially if there are arrows indicating that the glucose is changing quickly or it is within the first 24 h of a sensor.

The sensors come with tape to stick them to the body. Some people sweat the tape off or the tape simply doesn't stick well, or the tape irritates the skin. Some people use special wipes on the skin to make it stickier or use over- or under-bandages to help hold the sensor or reduce the contact with the skin. In most cases these issues can be overcome, but it often requires trial and error. The sensor companies can be helpful, as well as blogs and websites from people who have similar issues.

The transmitter is attached to the sensor to send the results to the receiver. Think of it like a walkie-talkie. The transmitter is generally small and in some cases rechargeable. Others lose their charge every 6–12 months and need to be replaced. Be careful not to throw out the transmitter along with the sensor. They are very expensive if they need to be replaced.

The receiver is the part of the system that displays the glucose levels and the trends and is where the setup for the CGM occurs. The receiver can vibrate or set off an alarm. Family members or friends can follow glucose levels on their smartphones. This can be very helpful, especially for children, whose parents want to be sure they are safe when they are at school or staying overnight with friends.

Uses of Sensor Data

Real-time analysis: Instead of a fingerstick done every few hours, these devices measure glucose level every 5 min. They can alert the wearer to a low blood glucose level when a threshold value is crossed and show trends and send out an alert if the blood glucose level is falling quickly. You/your child will need a different dose of insulin if the blood glucose level is 100 mg/dL and going up compared with 100 mg/dL and going down quickly. This greater knowledge can help you/your child treat low blood glucose reactions sooner. It can also alert family members to an impending problem, particularly a low blood glucose level that requires corrective action.

Retrospective analysis: People using devices should upload the data to an appropriate website. The data can then be shared with the health-care team in between visits, especially if there are problems with diabetes management. And of course this is very useful during clinic visits.

> Look for patterns of low blood glucose reactions, so these can be corrected.

Look at your/your child's data every week or two. Look for patterns of low blood glucose reactions so that they can be corrected. Then high blood glucose levels can be addressed and doses can be adjusted. Variables such as days of the week (weekends vs. weekdays) as well as the effects of exercise can all be assessed and managed if problems exist.

Children: The Dexcom CGM is approved by the FDA down to the age of 2 years, the Medtronic Enlite CGM is approved for individuals aged >16 years, and the Medtronic 670G is approved for those aged >14 years. Regardless, many families who have an infant find using a CGM very helpful. Infants often can't communicate that they are feeling unwell, so CGMs can be invaluable in detecting low blood glucose. Getting insurance companies to pay for CGMs in this age group can be very challenging. Even if your child is in an FDA-approved age group, insurance approval can be challenging and varies a lot between insurance providers. Medicaid typically does not cover CGMs; however, this is changing. Insurance companies are more likely to approve CGMs in children who have frequent low glucose levels, severe low glucose reactions, unawareness of their low glucose levels, or highly variable glucose levels.

Adults: For many adults, CGM devices can be obtained through health insurance. CGM systems that can be used to make treatment decisions have recently been classified as durable medical equipment under Medicare Part B. Medicare covers one type of CGM for certain individuals with diabetes and a few states cover CGM for adults on Medicaid. Rates of severe hypoglycemia increase with age. For those who can't afford to get a CGM, frequent fingerstick checking is the alternative.

Abbondanza!

"Cinque Terre is a gorgeous chain of five cliffside towns that overlook the Italian Riviera. Full of working vineyards and quaint stone farmhouses, it is a postcard-perfect UNESCO-protected slice of heaven. But lurking in paradise was poison. Italy is a country awash in carbs: pizza carbs, pasta carbs, pastry carbs, risotto carbs, gelato carbs.

Before my trip, my Endo suggested I consider a brand new technology: a continuous glucose monitor. 'It's like a Nintendo. It makes following your numbers like a video game.' I wasn't a gamer and the idea of being constantly attached to another device was so, uh, juvenile. 'I'll think about it,' I said flatly and promptly rejected the advice

The 3-h hike across the thin mountain paths that connect the five towns of Cinque Terre was challenging. I was tired, thirsty, and possibly sporting low BG numbers, but had left my 'stick-and-read' meter and strips at the hotel. Happily, everything was well within range that very evening after my trek and an Italian dinner that proudly proclaimed abbondanza!

But at 3 a.m., something was clearly wrong. I awoke with the rapid heartbeat, the cold sweats, the disorientation. Whether I was still dreaming or hallucinating, I thought I was 'going towards the light.'

My BG was 38, an all-time low. With that, I attacked the minibar and vacuumed down every juice, soda, and candy bar I could find. Eventually the terror subsided enough that I could contact my doctor and ask for answers. She told me what to do and said, 'Come in and see me when you're back.'

So I did. And soon afterwards, I relented and got my first CGM. And became completely dependent on its early warning alerts. I've worn it every single day for 11 years and could not survive without it. It was expensive, bulky, and yet another thing to carry along with my iPhone, wallet, keys, and sunglasses. But the volume of information it provided to both me and my Endo proved invaluable, the intrusive high and low alerts it emits at all hours of the day or night lifesaving.

Since then, I've preached the gospel of CGM to every newly diagnosed diabetic that has yet to accept CGM into his or her life. Yes, it could be improved—thank heavens it now talks directly to my iPhone!—but it is a unique and highly dependable 24/7 weapon in my 24/7 battle against diabetes.

Better still: I know I can return to Italy without fear of abbondanza. And THAT's postcard-perfect!"

—Neil Newman, 57, is a marketing and sales consultant.

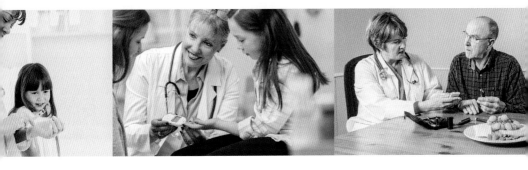

CHAPTER 4

The Diabetes Team

There is incredibly good news about having type 1 diabetes—it is a treatable condition. People are now living long, healthy, and active lives with diabetes. Advances in treatments and technologies have helped cause these improvements, but it is the people with diabetes themselves who have learned how to use these treatments and improve their health. We know now what it takes to live a long life with diabetes.

The bad news is that diabetes management falls on the person with the disease and their family and caregivers. It requires daily attention to detail and management. Diabetes burnout is discussed in Chapter 9. The key to getting the right care is creating the right health-care team and getting the assistance you/your child needs. This can be one of the most difficult challenges in dealing with diabetes. Sometimes this challenge is easier for children because there are large pediatric diabetes programs around the country. Adults, on the other hand, may not be able to find a specialist in type 1 diabetes. It is perhaps hardest of all for people between the ages of 18 and 30 years who are in transition from one form of care to another.

Look What You Can Do

"I remember my first diabetes doctor. He was old and mean. He was upset that my honeymoon period was over and I was having a lot of trouble controlling my blood sugars. My A1C was around 12. He told me, 'You're not going to die, you know?! You're going to go blind, or lose a leg, or ugh!' And then he walked out of the room. Shortly after, we looked for a new doctor. That's when I found the team I have been with ever since. They tried a few things to get me to turn my life around. Eventually, it worked. My A1C is now 6.2. When I see my doctor, she says with a smile, 'Look at that, give you a few tools and look at what you can do.' I am so thankful for her and my nurse practitioner/diabetes educator."

—Amirah Meghani

JUST DIAGNOSED

The experience of a person who is in the hospital at the beginning of their diabetes versus someone who is just diagnosed as part of their routine medical follow-up is very different. But what is needed for all is to find a health-care provider knowledgeable in diabetes who can lead your team.

> **Whether young or old, requiring hospitalization for new-onset diabetes can be traumatizing.**

Getting the best care begins on day 1 of a type 1 diabetes diagnosis, or when you go to a new health-care provider for the first time. The initial assessment is your opportunity to tell the provider who you/your child/your family is: your medical history, your experiences, and your beliefs.

Starting in the Hospital

Whether young or old, requiring hospitalization for new-onset diabetes can be traumatizing. You/your child might be very ill, with symptoms of out-of-control diabetes such as excessive thirst, dehydration, frequent urination, weight loss, headache, abdominal pain, rapid and shallow respirations, or even coma. Generally, this leads to a mad rush to the emergency room and an admission to the intensive care unit.

Sometimes a child may be thirsty and urinating frequently but otherwise well. The child may still require hospitalization so that the parents can learn how to manage diabetes. This can be incredibly disorienting—to find yourself or your child seriously ill and find out that the problem is the chronic, lifelong disease that is type 1 diabetes. Everyone has a different reaction, from the person with the diagnosis to their friends and family. Parents who need to be responsible to care for their child have a unique set of concerns; the spouse of someone newly diagnosed has another. Regardless, there are four things to remember and repeat:

1.   It will get better.
2.   You will adjust.
3.   You are not alone.
4.   It is not your fault.

There are many people who you will seek out to help you on your diabetes journey: doctors, diabetes educators, nurses and nurse practitioners, school nurses, physician assistants, pharmacists, dietitians, medical assistants, and perhaps a counselor, to name a few. A neighbor or a friend with type 1 diabetes can be very helpful.

In addition to organizations such as the ADA and JDRF, there are some wonderful bloggers and groups of people with diabetes who connect and help each other. Be careful of some of the information you receive. Some of the bloggers and even at times some companies looking to sell you things are wrong, inappropriately negative, even scary, or they promise their technology or drug can do something to help you with your diabetes that it cannot do. See the **Appendix** for organizations we recommend.

But back to the hospital. Usually in the hospital the goal is to treat whatever is making you/your child so sick—often people have DKA—and then give you the basic survival skills to manage your diabetes outside the hospital until you meet with your new diabetes management team. The usual way to treat DKA is to give fluids and insulin through your veins in order to return the body to a safe range. Giving insulin intravenously usually means time spent in or near an intensive care unit because more nursing time and supervision is needed.

Once you/your child can eat and drink fluids again, usually within a day or two, you (adult) or your parents (child) will learn how to give shots and the basics of living with diabetes. There should also be meetings with a dietitian to learn about nutrition and how food and insulin relate to each other.

Realize that this is a crash course—just survival skills. Over the next weeks and months, more complete learning happens. Don't feel like you need to learn everything all at once.

Often the insulin doses started in the hospital will change, usually becoming less, over the next few weeks at home. Be prepared to contact your healthcare provider often to make adjustments. This is a situation in which it is fine—encouraged, in fact—to call your diabetes team often. You aren't supposed to know this all on your own. Lean on your team to help you through every step.

While learning in the hospital, be sure to do the following:

1. Take notes, many notes. Your memory won't be as sharp as usual. If you are not feeling well enough or feel overwhelmed, ask a trusted family member or friend.
2. Ask questions—there is no such thing as a stupid question.
3. Don't be upset with yourself for not learning quickly—generally people are a bit in shock and it is hard to learn when stunned.
4. Write down questions that occur to you after the diabetes team member has gone.
5. Avoid excessive reliance on the Internet for information. Each person with diabetes is different, and there are too many worst-case scenarios to be found. You are going to be a best-case scenario.
6. Especially in the case of a child, ask all care providers, including grandparents, aunts and uncles, babysitters, or nannies, to participate in the education if they spend a lot of time with your child.

When you leave the hospital, be sure that you have the following:

1. All the diabetes supplies you need, including insulin. It is a good idea to get all of the prescriptions filled and bring them to the hospital for your diabetes team to check.
2. Prescriptions called into your pharmacy that include insulin, blood test strips, pen needles or needles and syringes, lancets, glucagon, ketone-testing strips, and glucose tabs/gel.
3. A contact number for the person(s) who will be helping adjust your/your child's insulin doses each day.
4. An appointment with an endocrinologist within the first month after discharge so that you can establish care.

THE INITIAL OUTPATIENT EXAM: GENERAL GUIDELINES

The first appointment with your/your child's new endocrinologist or diabetes health-care provider should be very thorough. You want to be fully checked out and have your needs and issues understood. Often this visit will be with the endocrinologist, certified diabetes educator (CDE), dietitian, and social worker or psychologist, so plan on spending a couple hours at the clinic. General ideas for what this checkup should look like are listed in the next section.

Diabetes Type

Children: Most children aged <10 years will have type 1 diabetes. For adolescents who could have type 2 diabetes, discuss diabetes type and be clear if it is type 1 or type 2. In Chapter 2, there are some suggestions as to how to figure out what type of diabetes your child has.

Adults: Make sure your doctor knows you have type 1 diabetes, not type 2, especially if you opt to go to a primary care or family doctor, who may have mostly patients with type 2 diabetes. If you don't know what type of diabetes you have, feel free to ask for clarification.

First Impressions

Briefly describe how and when diabetes was diagnosed and all prior treatment. What happened at your initial diagnosis? Did you go to the hospital? Were your symptoms mild or severe? How old were you?

Children: For children who can talk, let them tell the health-care provider about their experience. It can help for parents and children to speak with a counselor separately if the first experience with diabetes was particularly stressful or difficult.

Adults: It is often helpful to briefly outline the main reason for your visit (such as a recent move and need to establish care with a new endocrinologist or because you are having diabetes issues that aren't being addressed by your prior doctor).

Personal History

This is where you/your child should summarize the past in terms of diabetes experiences. Most important is what has gone well as well as what hasn't worked.

Children: Tell everything about your child's life with diabetes, including school and caregivers, activities and exercise habits, eating patterns, relationships, and everything that seems pertinent to incorporating diabetes management into your child's life. This will be age-specific—the concerns of a parent with a toddler will be very different from those of a parent of an adolescent. Much of this part of the visit may be with a certified diabetes educator, a registered dietitian, or a counselor. The more you tell a doctor about your concerns and observations (and have your child speak as well), the better. For older children, speaking with the health-care provider privately without a parent present may be helpful. This should be based on your child's comfort with the new health-care setting. Ask about diabetes support groups and local diabetes summer camps that the clinic may be associated with, because it is helpful to meet other people living with diabetes.

Adults: Briefly summarize the past experiences you have had living with diabetes. You may be able to provide insight as to what didn't work in the past—for instance that you tried a pump or sensor and then stopped wearing it. You can talk about the various phases of your life and how diabetes has impacted you. More specific questions to answer include: Have you been hospitalized in the past? Do you have any complications, including acute complications such as diabetic ketoacidosis, or chronic complications such as eye disease? Are you having tingling in your hands or feet? Are you having trouble with frequent, mild low blood glucose reactions? Do you have a history of having severe low blood glucose reactions in which you passed out, had a seizure, or needed help from someone else to get glucose?

Family History

Anyone else in the family have diabetes? Type 1 and/or 2? Thyroid, celiac disease, adrenal disease, or vitiligo? What about heart disease, high blood pressure, or kidney disease? Cancer? Rheumatoid arthritis, lupus, multiple sclerosis? Anything else?

> Health-care providers are only as helpful as the data they are given—minimal data, minimal advice.

Current Treatment

Bring all diabetes pieces to the exam: meter(s), pump, sensor, home and school logs, insulin pens and vials. The more you bring to your health-care providers, the more help you/your child can receive. Health-care providers are only as helpful as the data they are given—minimal data, minimal advice. Use them to the fullest. Bring data! Mention whether or not you are satisfied with your current plan, and be specific. If you're not happy with some aspect of your care or the care your child is receiving, maybe it's time for a change.

Questions and Concerns

Bring a list of questions. If you are new to diabetes, prepare to take notes and ask for printed materials. Learning new concepts takes multiple repetitions—ask, and ask again, until you are sure of the answer.

There is no question that is too stupid to ask if it is something unanswered. Fears about other family members, particularly siblings or children, developing type 1 diabetes are common. Cost issues are real and insurance companies can make getting the right supplies and medications difficult. These concerns should be addressed with your health-care team as well.

Children: Parents, don't be afraid to ask questions. Type 1 is tricky and getting comfortable is key for not only health and safety but also for peace of mind. Having a young child develop a chronic disease can be devastating and is bound to affect your emotional state. Feelings of guilt, fear, and frustration are completely normal. Explore these issues with your provider and get whatever support you need.

Adults: It may take a while to trust and open up to a new provider, especially if you've been followed by a pediatrician you are particularly fond of. Many issues, new and old, face adults with type 1 diabetes. In addition to the usual issues with blood glucose management, there may be concerns about drinking alcohol or using marijuana, relationships and sex, erectile dysfunction and loss of libido, having children, fighting workplace discrimination, dealing with medical costs, and all the other issues of adulthood. Some of these are directly medical, others are more psychosocial, and all can impact blood glucose levels. Not all may come up at the first visit but can hopefully be addressed over time.

Medical Nutrition Therapy

Diabetes requires a solid education in balancing carbs, insulin, and exercise. Ask for a referral to a diabetes educator and a dietitian. This is helpful at diagnosis and at intervals along the way. Never stop being a learner or asking for help.

The Physical Exam

The provider should perform a thorough evaluation of you/your child's current health, looking for any diabetes complications or additional autoimmune disorders (celiac disease, thyroid disease, etc.), usually done through some blood tests. **Table 10.1** in Chapter 10 lists the recommendations for the blood and urine tests that should be done at least once a year. Remember to get and keep copies of these! You need to start a file and be a little bit of a pack rat. Keep all of the lab and other medical reports and compare them each time new ones are taken. Look for changes and abnormal values and ask your health-care provider if they mean anything important.

In terms of the examination, at a minimum the provider should check blood pressure and pulse, examine the thyroid, heart, lungs, and abdomen, and look at the insulin injection or infusion sites to be sure they are not inflamed, infected, or overused.

Children: The provider will measure your child's height and weight and may also need to examine your child to see where he or she is in puberty, as knowing this will help them make insulin dose adjustments. Your child's diabetes provider may not be the same person as his or her regular pediatrician, so if there are issues or concerns from either provider, they need to communicate about your child's care.

Adults: In adults, your doctor should also do a complete foot exam and then repeat it at every visit if there are any potential problems. This generally means looking at the foot and between the toes, testing for sensation, checking reflexes, pulses, and nails, and looking for deformities of the feet and any evidence of an infection.

Making a Plan

Now that your doctor knows you/your child, it's time to establish how you're going to be taking care of yourself until your next visit and what to do in case of an emergency. This plan is flexible and will change over time as you enter into various stages of diabetes life and life in general. It is best to have this as a written plan, including a complete list of your local resources, how to contact the clinic, and how to get after-hours help. You need to know whom to contact for prescriptions and prior authorizations for medications and diabetes devices, and to fill out paperwork for attending school or going to camp. Be sure you know how much lead time is needed for prescriptions, especially if you use mail order. Leave your clinic visit with a diabetes plan for sick days and exercise days as well. Always best to be prepared!

> Leave your clinic visit with a diabetes plan for sick days and exercise days as well.

Centered around You/Your Child

The diabetes care provided to you/your child should be patient-centered because you will be happier and healthier if you have a voice in your care or the care of your child. You, as patient or the parent of a patient, are in a partnership with your health-care providers. Together, this team tackles the tough questions such as what blood glucose goals are right for you/your child and whether you'd do better with a pump. Putting the patient at the center of the equation ensures that whatever your/your child's individual quirks—a love of ballet, a fondness for cookies, a favorite sports team, or a goal of climbing Kilimanjaro—you/your child will get individualized care.

> You must be the advocate for yourself or your child. No one else will care as much as you do.

Not all providers are familiar with the patient-centered approach. You as the patient have the right to assert yourself. It's your life; make sure you share with your doctor how you want to live it. You must be the advocate for yourself or your child. No one else will care as much as you do.

Beware of providers you feel are judgmental or unwilling to listen to your/your child's needs. Blood glucose levels are not "good" or "bad," and the provider should both cheer progress and accept imperfection. Shame and blame should not be a part of a visit with your diabetes team.

A good idea is to formulate one goal at each visit to work on before the next visit. That goal can be as simple as to exercise 4 days per week instead of 2 or to reduce after-dinner snacking to lower late-evening blood glucose levels. It is too generic to say, "In 3 months, I want to have a fall in A1C from 8% to 7%." That is a great goal, but it is more helpful to identify specific action steps, such as checking more blood glucose levels or reducing overnight high blood glucose levels. Then create a plan that leads to that goal.

Goals

"At the age of 40, I strive to achieve the goals I set for myself. I am blessed to work with a great diabetes team. The team and I are working on more consistent blood glucose testing, especially first thing in the morning and before bed. I sometimes struggle with laziness and feeling I can cheat my way through this intricate part of care. I don't have an updated computer, so we set a goal for me to upload my readings on another machine. The achievement of this goal will help me to achieve my big goal: an A1C of 7.0 or lower.

I often consider the fact that diabetes is not a result of anything I did or did not do, that it didn't appear in the lineage of either side of my family until after I was diagnosed. When I look back over my life I can honestly say that anything I ever wanted to do, I was able to do it: run track, be a high school cheerleader, travel, participate in a step competition with my sorority, and live independently. I think it's safe to say, I have diabetes, but it doesn't have me."

— Roberta Sonsaray White, M.Div., is a chaplain in the health-care setting.

Primary care provider: This can be an internist, pediatrician, family practitioner, nurse practitioner, or physician assistant, among others. In many settings your primary care provider is different from the endocrinologist who follows your diabetes, although in some cases this is the same person. The primary care provider is generally the person who coordinates all of your care from various specialists. If you need a basic checkup or get sick, a primary care provider is the person to go to first. In some health-care systems, you are required to have a primary care provider to refer you to an endocrinologist; with other types of insurance this may not be necessary.

Endocrinologist: These specialists focus on the endocrine system, which includes the hormones that keep your body functioning properly and the glands that make those hormones. Diabetes falls under the endocrine umbrella because it's a disorder of insulin, a hormone. Endocrinologists also take care of people with thyroid disorders, which are more common in people with type 1 diabetes. Many people with type 1 see an endocrinologist, especially when first diagnosed or if they are having challenges with care. Children almost always see a pediatric endocrinologist; adults may or may not be able to find an endocrinologist in their area. What matters is that the care provided is high quality and healthy A1C and other health goals are being supported and met.

Certified diabetes educator: People with a specific degree (such as an RN, NP, or RD) and a special interest in diabetes can become CDEs. They are basically diabetes tutors. They help you learn how to do the many complex diabetes tasks. CDEs must pass a national test every 5 years that covers physiology, medications, blood glucose monitoring, complications, mental health issues, and teaching/learning principles.

Registered dietitian: A registered dietitian with expertise in diabetes will teach you how to count carbs, cover high-fat meals, figure in special treats, how to safely enjoy alcohol, match food with physical activity and insulin, lose or gain weight if needed, or follow a gluten-free diet if you have celiac disease.

Eye doctor: This is either an ophthalmologist or an optometrist who is familiar with eye disease in people with diabetes and can do the recommended testing.

Mental health expert: Diabetes distress can affect both the person with diabetes and caregivers. Social workers, psychologists, psychiatrists, and family therapists can help a person with type 1 and their families navigate the emotional and psychological aspects of living with a chronic disease.

Podiatrist: Diabetes can damage the blood vessels and nerves, particularly in the feet. Prevention and early intervention are critical for maintaining foot health. A podiatrist can help you learn about foot care and how to spot problems. Foot sores and calluses require a trip to a diabetes-friendly podiatrist; don't try to treat them yourself. Ask your diabetes doctor if you need to see a podiatrist.

Pharmacist: A pharmacist can tell you about side effects and drug interactions. Sticking with one pharmacy is helpful: they'll have a record of all the medications you take and can alert you to any red flags. Pharmacists are also experts in over-the-counter medications and can guide you toward diabetes-friendly options. A pharmacist can be your ally in getting approval from your health insurance company for various medications and supplies. This process is known as "prior authorization" and means that the medication you/your child needs isn't routinely covered under your insurance, but if your pharmacy or healthcare provider gives enough information to justify it, then you can get the medication needed.

Dentist: Going to the dentist every 6 months for a checkup and a cleaning is a good idea for everyone, but especially for people with diabetes. Type 1 diabetes increases the risk of gum disease. Make sure your dentist knows you/your child has diabetes.

Exercise physiologist: An exercise physiologist can design a physical activity plan that takes into account any of your physical limitations and incorporates strategies to avoid blood glucose going too low.

Other specialists: Older adults may need to see other specialists, such as cardiologists, nephrologists, and neurologists.

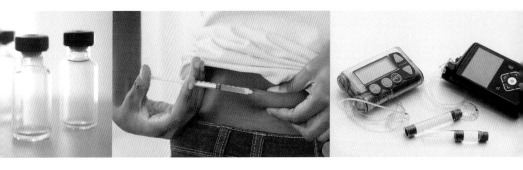

CHAPTER 5

Insulin and Delivery Devices

Insulin is a hormone, meaning it gets made in one part of the body, in this case the pancreas, and travels to other parts of the body to do a job. Insulin attaches to receptors on the surface of muscle and fat cells. Once insulin is bound, the cell responds by opening up tiny doors in its outer layer or membrane, which allows glucose from the blood to flow into the cell.

> Insulin release from a nondiabetic pancreas is a finely tuned process, and levels increase and decrease based on signals from many parts of the body, including the brain.

In those without diabetes, specialized cells in the pancreas, called β-cells, deliver a steady low-level stream of insulin, called "basal" or "background" insulin. The β-cells also release larger amounts of insulin in response to food intake, stress, and certain medications, among other triggers. The insulin is released in little tiny pulses or bursts that overlap, creating a smooth effect, rather than in larger "bolus" doses as is given by people with diabetes.

Once the insulin is released, some is swept up into the liver, where it works to balance the liver's use of glucose. Sometimes the liver releases glucose and sometimes it stores glucose. After working on the liver, the insulin circulates to all other parts of the body. Some of the insulin escapes extraction by the liver and directly reaches peripheral tissues. Insulin release from a nondiabetic pancreas is a finely tuned process, and levels increase and decrease based on signals from many parts of the body, including the brain.

The insulin-producing β-cells live within islets of Langerhans, clusters of cells that make up 1–2% of the pancreas and looked to their discoverer, Paul Langerhans, like little islands on a pancreatic sea, hence the name. Alongside the β-cells, the islets store α-cells, which make glucagon. This hormone is basically anti-insulin, raising blood glucose instead of lowering it. The β- and α-cells listen to each other, releasing their respective hormones at different times. The release of insulin from β-cells indicates that the body is well supplied with glucose, and the insulin acts as a signal to the α-cells not to release glucagon. A dip in insulin means there may be a shortage of glucose in the blood, and alerts the α-cells that they should bring glucose levels up by releasing glucagon.

> Glucagon is basically anti-insulin, raising blood glucose instead of lowering it.

MEET TEAM INSULIN

Insulin delivered subcutaneously (under the skin) from a syringe or pump doesn't work as well as the insulin made by the body. However, scientists con-

TABLE 5.1   Insulins on the Market

Type of insulin	Brand name (generic name)	Starts working	Works hardest	Stops working
Background *Long-acting*	Lantus (U100 glargine) Basaglar (U100 biosimilar glargine) Toujeo (U300 glargine) Levemir (detemir)	2 h	Steady most of the day	14–24 h
Background *Ultralong-acting*	Tresiba (U100 or U200) (degludec)		Steady	~42 h
Background *Intermediate-acting, NPH*	Humulin N Novolin N Novolin/ReliOn N	2–4 h	4–8 h	10–16 h
Mealtime *Rapid-acting*	Apidra (glulisine) Humalog (lispro) NovoLog (aspart)	15 min	1–2 h	3–4 h
Mealtime *Short-acting, regular*	Humulin R Novolin R Novolin/ReliOn R	30–45 min	2–3 h	4–8 h
Mealtime *Ultra-rapid-acting*	Afrezza (inhaled) fiasp (aspart)	0–10 min 5–15 min	1 h 1–3 h	2–3 h 3–4 h
Premixed *Intermediate-acting/rapid-acting*	Humalog Mix 75/25 Humalog Mix (50/50) Novolog Mix (70/30)	15 min	1–2 h	10–16 h
Premixed *Intermediate-acting/regular*	Humulin 70/30 Novolin 70/30 Novolin ReliOn 70/30	30–45 min	2–3 h	10–16 h

tinue to make improvements, and there are a variety of insulin types on the market **(Table 5.1)**.

Most people with type 1 diabetes who use injections need to take two types of insulin: a long-acting insulin for basal (background) coverage and a short- or rapid-acting insulin to cover meals. People who use insulin pumps use one type of insulin.

Older Insulins

Regular insulin and NPH insulin have been on the market for many years. Regular insulin is also referred to as a short-acting insulin, while NPH is sometimes called an intermediate-acting insulin.

These older insulins are less expensive than newer insulins. But they can be difficult to match to the body's insulin needs. Regular insulin usually needs to be given at least 15–30 min before eating. These medications tend to be more variable in the body (meaning the effect of any given dose is less easy to predict) and can cause more low blood glucose reactions. They also mimic natural insulin secretion less well; when injected under the skin, regular insulin takes longer to start working and lasts longer than insulin that comes from the pancreas. NPH insulin has a peak of activity somewhere from 6 to 12 h after it is injected, so it is not a good long-acting insulin.

If you work with a diabetes team familiar with their use, it is possible to manage type 1 diabetes with these older, much less expensive insulins. However, it is more of a challenge. Newer insulins are preferred for the treatment of type 1 diabetes, if possible.

Newer Insulins

Newer insulins have some advantages, such as being more reliable and predictable in terms of how they act and causing fewer low blood glucose reactions.

Basal or Long-Acting Insulin (Glargine, Detemir, and Degludec)

Basal insulin sticks around the body for a while, mimicking the low and constant insulin presence observed in people without diabetes. Basal insulin helps keep glucose in the target range between meals and prevents the liver, the body's glucose storehouse and manufacturing plant, from releasing excess glucose into the blood. Their effectiveness tends to be measured by the fasting, or before-breakfast, blood glucose level. Depending on the person and his or her response to the insulin, glargine and detemir may be given once or twice a day (morning and/or evening), whereas degludec is always given once a day. Ultralong-acting degludec causes fewer low blood glucose reactions, specifically nocturnal reactions, than glargine and may help provide a less variable basal insulin than seen with others on the market. The downside is that it should only be adjusted every 2 to 3 days, unlike glargine or detemir, which can be adjusted on a daily basis.

Prandial (Mealtime), Rapid-Acting (Lispro, Aspart, Glulisine), or Ultra-Rapid-Acting Insulin (fiasp)

Rapid-acting insulins are made for fast absorption in an attempt to imitate the bursts of insulin the β-cells release as a meal is absorbed, so they manage the postmeal peak glucose level. These insulin types are also broken down fairly quickly in the body, lowering the risk of hypoglycemia in the hours after a meal. They are usually given either immediately before a meal or 10–20 min in advance, depending on the blood glucose level. Sometimes people give them after eating if they have difficulty being sure that they will be able to eat all of their meal, or they give ~50% of the dose before the meal and then give the appropriate remainder when the meal is finished and the total carbohydrate consumption is known. This strategy can be helpful with small children and seniors who are having challenges eating. These are the insulins that are used in insulin pumps.

Premixed Insulins

In premixed insulins, part of the insulin is long-acting and part is short- or rapid-acting. Premixed insulins are generally not preferred because the ratios of shorter- to longer-acting insulin are fixed—you can't, say, give more short-acting insulin because the blood glucose is higher or more carbohydrates will be eaten. But for some people, in some settings, these insulins are helpful. It all comes back to the team and what works best for you/your child.

Inhaled Insulin

Inhaled insulin is absorbed through the lungs. Afrezza rapid-acting insulin comes in a small, purple, handheld inhaler. It is a powder that works even more rapidly than rapid-acting insulin and also stops working more quickly. It must be used along with a long-acting insulin in people with type 1 diabetes. Smokers and those with asthma or other lung problems should not use inhaled insulin. Afrezza is not yet approved for children; however, studies are underway. The smallest amount that can be delivered in an inhaler is too much for most children.

WHERE TO GIVE INSULIN

Insulin should be given into what is called the subcutaneous (SQ) tissue. This is so the insulin can be slowly absorbed into the bloodstream. If it is given into the muscle or a blood vessel, it will act much more quickly. In general, the needles for giving insulin make sure that it goes into the SQ tissue and nowhere else. Sometimes people worry about hitting the wrong place—maybe an organ or a bone or somewhere insulin doesn't belong. But this isn't possible with the small needles that are used for injecting insulin **(Fig. 5.1)**.

Shots can be given by the person with diabetes or their caregiver. Although for small children injections are almost always given by someone else, this can even be a sign of affection in older people as well. Some adult patients prefer to

Where to Give Insulin

- Abdomen: To inject in the abdomen (stomach), stay 2 inches away from the belly button or any scars you may have. Tip: Make a fist and place it over the belly button and inject anywhere else in the abdomen.
- Upper outer thigh: Inject one hand's width above the knee and one hand's width down from the top of the leg. Avoid injecting in the inner thigh due to large number of blood vessels and nerves in that area.
- Buttocks: Avoid the lower portion.
- Back of arms: Injecting into the arm may be difficult. Apply pressure to the arm from a fixed surface to create an injection site and then use a free hand to inject.

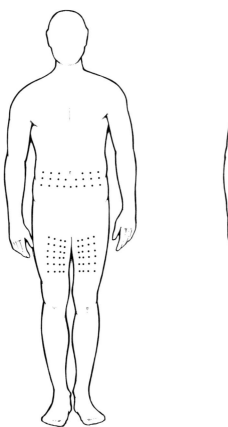
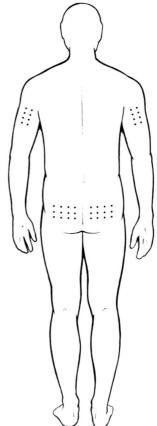

FIGURE 5.1   Injection sites.

Source: *Diabetes A to Z*, 7th edition. Alexandria, VA, American Diabetes Association, 2016, p. 88.

have their spouses involved in giving injections. Whatever works to make living with type 1 diabetes easier.

> Overall injections should be fairly painless, although occasionally a nerve under the skin is irritated, which can hurt but doesn't mean anything serious.

There are differing recommendations about pinching up the skin for giving the shot. With the shorter needles it isn't needed, but with longer needles it is. Children or very lean adults may also require that the skin is pinched up, so ask someone on your diabetes team what is recommended. If you use 4-mm pen needles, you do not need to pinch up the skin. If you/your child is lean, you may need to pinch up the skin if using 5-mm pen needles or 6-mm syringe needles. If you use needles 8-mm or longer, pinch up the skin. As long as the needle goes under the skin and the insulin is pushed in, it will work. Pushing the needle in fast is often less painful than going in slowly. Overall injections should be fairly painless, although occasionally a nerve under the skin is irritated, which can hurt but doesn't mean anything serious.

Sometimes bruising at the injection sites can happen. This is not serious and the insulin is still working. However, people who take aspirin or other medications to thin the blood will have more bruising than others. Also, older people with thinner skin may bruise more easily. Unfortunately there is no good way to avoid this, but rotating injection sites remains the best way to keep the area healthy and ensure that insulin is absorbed evenly.

> If insulin is given at the same site over and over again, scar tissue can build up.

If insulin is given at the same site over and over again, scar tissue can build up. This is known as lipohypertrophy. This is because insulin makes the fat cells grow. These areas become less painful for injecting; however, they need to be avoided because 1) insulin is absorbed erratically from these areas, sometimes too quickly and sometimes too slowly, which can make blood glucose levels more variable, and 2) these sites only keep growing and can look unsightly.

The way to cure this problem is to avoid injecting in the area until it has returned to normal. Some people have used microliposuction to get rid of some of the excess fat.

Syringes

The original insulin delivery system, syringes are still an option for people with diabetes. You'll need a syringe with needle attached and an insulin vial. Insulin is drawn from the vial into the syringe by tipping the insulin bottle upside down and pulling the plunger until the proper dose is achieved. Generally, some air is injected into the vial first in order not to create a vacuum.

There are three dimensions to any syringe-needle system. First, the size of the syringe. Syringes can be 1cc, 1/2cc, and 1/3cc. Having a syringe that is the right size makes it easier to see the lines to measure the insulin. And it is less clumsy to use. Second, there is the length of the needle, with ranges from shorter to longer. Third, there is the size of the needle (how big around it is). The smallest pen needles are 32 gauge (a large number means a smaller needle size). Most syringe needles are a bit bigger although generally the smaller the gauge (the larger the number) the less the pain. Finally, there are 1/3cc syringes with half-unit markings that may be needed by people taking very small, exacting doses of insulin.

Figure out which needle system is best for you/your child and then make sure your health-care provider orders it. It's helpful to have a CDE watch your injection technique or make a recommendation about which needle system might work best for you. If it hurts less and is easier to use, then you should have it! But you may need to bring in a needle package as a "show and tell" so your doctor can copy it exactly onto your next prescription. Physicians may not always know which diabetes supplies you prefer and we want to get it right! So help us order exactly what works best for you.

Pens

Insulin pens combine the medication and syringe in one convenient package. Pens come in two basic types: disposable and reusable. Disposable pens are preloaded with insulin and are discarded after the insulin cartridge is empty or the pen has been in use for 28 or 32 days (depending on insulin type). Reusable pens work with insulin cartridges that can be loaded into the pen and then tossed away once the insulin is used, leaving the pen ready for the next cartridge. Some pens dose in half-unit increments (e.g., 1.5 units), while others dose in whole units. This may be a consideration for people who are very sensitive to insulin, such as children and lean adults. The maximum dosage of insulin that can be delivered at one time also varies among pens.

Pen Needle Pointers

As with the needles on syringes, pen needles vary in terms of length and gauge. A higher gauge means a thinner needle. The length of the needles varies from 4 to 13 mm, and people often have very specific preferences as to the needle size they prefer. All of the pen needles work to deliver insulin, although sometimes too long a needle may lead to an injection into muscle in a lean person. Because this will change how the insulin acts, this is another area in which talking with your diabetes team can be useful. If you are particularly nervous about injections, there are also "shielded" needles so that you don't have to see the actual needle at all.

Be sure to prime the pen before you use it. Squirt out a unit or two of insulin straight up into the air once you put a new needle on. This makes sure the system is working and there is no air in the needle. People often worry if they see a drop of insulin on the skin or some insulin that comes back out after an injection is given. Generally this is not something to worry about unless the dose is very small, but it helps to hold the needle under the skin for ~10 sec to be sure that all the insulin is given.

STARTING AND USING INSULIN INJECTIONS

Infants

When an infant is first diagnosed and started on insulin injections, they are usually started on multiple shots a day. Infants diagnosed at this age have a rapidly progressing form of type 1 diabetes and often do not have many functioning β-cells left at diagnosis. They need basal insulin plus rapid-acting insulin for their meals.

Find a pediatric diabetes center experienced in the management of infants with type 1 diabetes, as infants have unique needs. Some infants, particularly those diagnosed under the age of 9 months, have a form of diabetes called neonatal diabetes that is not autoimmune and requires a different evaluation and treatment.

Many pediatric diabetes centers use insulin pumps in infants very soon after if not at diagnosis so that very small insulin doses can be delivered. Some pediatric diabetes centers also teach parents to dilute the insulin so that very tiny doses can be accurately given. Most pediatric diabetes centers will admit an infant with newly diagnosed diabetes to the hospital for initiation of insulin and for diabetes education.

Children

When a child starts on insulin injections, they usually require multiple shots per day, unless they are diagnosed very early in the process and still have β-cells making insulin. If your child is in diabetic ketoacidosis, then they will be admitted to the hospital for intravenous insulin and fluids and then transitioned to SQ insulin and subsequent education. If your child is not in DKA, then they will either be admitted to the hospital for insulin initiation and education or this may be done in the outpatient clinic setting. Different pediatric diabetes centers do this differently, and either approach is fine. The decision to admit to the hospital or not is individualized for each child and their family's needs.

Adults

When an adult starts on insulin injections, they may need only one shot a day at first or require multiple shots. It all depends on how quickly the β-cells are losing the ability to make insulin and whether they have been treated as someone with type 2 diabetes initially, rather than someone with type 1 diabetes. Therefore, some adults with new-onset type 1 diabetes may be in the hospital, where they are taught how to give insulin injections, but others will learn in their doctor's office.

> If you are an adult diagnosed with type 2 diabetes but you think you might have type 1 diabetes, you can ask to be tested for type 1 diabetes.

If you are an adult diagnosed with type 2 diabetes but you think you might have type 1 diabetes (e.g., you are lean, have no family history of type 2 diabetes, and/or are not responding to the type 2 diabetes medications you are given), you can ask to be tested for type 1 diabetes (see Chapter 2 for antibody tests). Sometimes you may find yourself educating your doctor, but it's important to find out what type of diabetes you have because it changes your treatment.

HOW TO TAKE INSULIN

Whether you are an adult or child, once your body stops making enough insulin to keep your blood glucose level in the target range before and after meals, you will need to give insulin in two different ways—as a basal dose (either by an injection of a long-acting insulin or through a pump, with its continuous flow of rapid-acting insulin) and bolus doses (rapid-acting insulin given by injection or through the pump).

The starting doses of basal and bolus insulin are usually determined based on weight. Often a slightly lower-than-calculated dose is started and gradually increased or decreased according to the response. Many factors go into determining the correct daily dose, and the dose required may change day to day based on physical activity and health. Over time, dose adjustments are often required and sometimes these doses become skewed—out of sync with what is the best insulin replacement program. Therefore, it is important to review the insulin dose program with your/your child's diabetes team to be sure the doses are correct.

Is Your Basal Dose Right?

The right dose of basal insulin will keep the blood glucose level roughly stable overnight (within 30–40 mg/dL from bedtime to wake-up time). If blood glucose increases >30 mg/dL overnight, an increase in basal may be needed, while a decrease of >30 mg/dL would indicate that basal should be lowered.

Insulin Pump Basal Rate

The insulin pump actually uses rapid-acting insulin to create basal insulin, delivering tiny pulses of insulin every few minutes 24 h a day. Rapid-acting insulin is more efficient than long-acting insulin, and so pump users usually need ~20% less basal insulin than those who use NPH or long-acting basal insulin.

> Unless you go through long periods of not eating during the day, the majority of the variability in daytime blood glucose levels will be due to the bolus insulin, not the basal rate.

Many people start off with a single basal rate, given as insulin units/hour, and then they fine-tune their basal rates to change throughout the day as their insulin needs vary. The daytime rate often differs from the nighttime rate. Again, use the 30-mg/dL yardstick. If your blood glucose increases >30 mg/dL during a period when you haven't eaten anything, increase basal slightly, and if it decreases >30 mg/dL, decrease basal slightly. Unless you go through long periods of not eating during the day, the majority of the variability in blood glucose levels will be due to the bolus insulin, not the basal rate. The basal effect will be most pronounced during the overnight period.

Optimizing basal rates on a pump can get complicated, so work with a CDE or pump trainer to help iron out all the kinks. If you're already using multiple daily injections, use your personalized total daily insulin dose to calculate your initial basal rate rather than a generic daily total calculated from your weight.

The 50:50 Principle of Insulin Management

Children: In children, basal insulin accounts for 25–50% of their total daily insulin. Infants and toddlers often need 25–30% of their total daily insulin as basal. As kids get older and approach puberty, their percent as basal insulin increases and approaches the need of adults, which is ~50% of the total daily insulin dose. Long-acting insulin is the preferred choice if you're not using a pump, and NPH is a backup if long-acting insulin is not an option.

Adults: Generally this ratio is 50:50, but it varies depending on the person and their circumstances. Occasionally, however, someone will have a high basal rate—totaling 80–90% of their daily insulin requirement. These individuals have to eat at regular intervals so as not to be driven too low by their basal insulin dose. If this works for an individual, then there may be no reason to change; however, many will end up gaining weight because they are eating for the insulin. Regardless, if the basal-to-bolus ratio is much different from 50:50 don't try to change to a more even ratio all at once. Small increments, with changes in both basal and bolus patterns, will bring the values into a better balance. And remember, if something is working correctly for you, you may not need to change it. Work with your health-care team to decide what is best.

Bolus Doses

The remainder of the total daily insulin dose is bolus insulin. Rapid-acting insulin, taken before meals and snacks, is the preferred choice, but short-acting regular insulin will do if rapid-acting insulin is not an option or if you/your child eats high-fat foods frequently. High-fat meals are absorbed more slowly and may best be covered by short-acting regular insulin, which has a longer duration of action than rapid-acting insulin.

> Rapid-acting insulin takes around 10–20 minutes to kick in, so for optimal timing, you'll want to pregame with insulin, and take it about 10–20 minutes before a meal or snack. Ultra-rapid-acting insulin will start acting sooner.

The premeal insulin amount is based on a carbohydrate dose plus a correction dose. Working with a dietitian and your diabetes provider is the best way to figure out the doses. Some people need the same amount of insulin for the carbs at different times of the day, and some people need more or less at the different meal times. For example, teenagers and adults typically need more insulin for the carbs at breakfast than later in the day, whereas school-aged children often need less insulin for lunch compared with the rest of the day.

For children, the insulin for carbs and correction depends on how much the child weighs and where they are in puberty. There is a large range and the dose needs to be individualized for each child.

Some people start with fixed doses that assume a fairly standard amount of carbohydrate with each meal. There are various formulas for determining these doses and they are different in children (where they are more specific) and in adults (where they tend to be more generic; also known as ballpark estimating).

Rapid-acting insulin takes ~10–20 min to kick in, so for optimal timing you'll want to pregame and take it ~10–20 min before a meal or snack. But be careful, once you take insulin, you need to eat to avoid a dangerous low. One good rule of thumb is that if your premeal glucose is in the 100s, take insulin 10 min before eating; if it is in the 200s, take insulin 20 min before eating; and if it is in the 300s, take insulin 30 min before eating.

The bolus component of the insulin regimen covers the rise in blood glucose that results from eating meals and snacks. Bolus doses need to be individualized to ensure that blood glucose doesn't go too high or too low. The main factors that determine bolus doses are as follows:

1.   Carbohydrate count.
2.   Current blood glucose level.
3.   Insulin remaining from previous boluses ("active insulin").
4.   Physical activity.
5.   The rate of change (a consideration for those who use CGM).

The basic bolus equation looks something like this:

$$\text{Bolus dose} = (\text{carbohydrate dose} + \text{correction dose} - \text{active insulin}) \times \text{physical activity adjustment}$$

> Each person has unique insulin needs, so the I:C is personal.

Insulin-to-Carb Ratio

Matching the amount of carbohydrate in a meal or snack to the bolus dose requires a conversion factor: your insulin-to-carb ratio (I:C). Each person has unique insulin needs, so the I:C is personal. The insulin-to-carb ratio is typically between 1:5 and 1:20 for adolescents and adults and between 1:10 and 1:40 for children. A good starting carb ratio for a relatively lean adult is 1:15 (1 unit of insulin for every 15 g of carbs eaten). However, these vary a lot and should be worked out with your health-care team. It may vary based on the time of day. Pumps can't tell if you are eating a high-fat meal. So sometimes you need to use different types of bolus doses, such as combination boluses (some up front, some later) or extended boluses (giving the bolus over time instead of all at once).

Active Insulin

Rapid-acting insulin typically stays in the body for 4–6 h, so there's likely to be some insulin left in your system if you eat meals or snacks <6 h apart. Insulin pumps calculate active insulin automatically and subtract it from the bolus dose. For those using injections, there are charts that calculate how much of your previous bolus has been used up based on how long it's been since that bolus. For example, if it's been 2 h since a bolus, 65% has been used up, so the active insulin would be 35% of that prior dose. This helps prevent something called "stacking," in which people give too much insulin too soon after the last dose, causing a low blood glucose reaction to occur.

Correction Dose

For this calculation, you'll need one more piece of the puzzle: your sensitivity factor or correction factor. This value estimates how much your blood glucose drops for every unit of bolus insulin you take. Sensitivity factors vary by person and time of day, so it will take some tinkering to find your personalized number.

In children, the starting dose is determined by body weight and where the child is in puberty. The starting number for a child can vary between 50 and >200.

Often we start with a number of 50 in adolescents and adults, which means 1 unit drops the blood glucose by 50 mg/dL. A thinner patient may have a correction of 100 and a heavier person a correction of 25. People often know this number intuitively if they have been on insulin for a while.

To calculate a correction dose you'll also need to know your current blood glucose as well as your target blood glucose: 150 mg/dL is a good place to start, but this may lower to 120 mg/dL as your diabetes becomes better managed. Example:

Glucose level before breakfast (current) = 220 mg/dL
Target blood glucose before meals = 120 mg/dL
Sensitivity factor = 44

The equation is as follows:

$$\text{Correction dose} = (\text{current glucose} - \text{target glucose})/\text{sensitivity factor}$$
$$(220 - 120)/44 = 2.27 \text{ or } \sim2 \text{ units of insulin}$$

Pumps also have the ability to subtract insulin if the blood glucose level is too low (or if there is active insulin, as noted previously).

Physical Activity Factor

If you're planning to go for a long run, mow the lawn, or engage in some other form of activity after a bolus, factor that into the dose. Activity acts like another insulin, lowering blood glucose in its own way. We'll cover this more in Chapter 7, but for now, just note that there are adjustments that should be made for exercise. These adjustments in insulin doses help protect against blood glucose lows. You may need to factor in physical activity that occurred before your bolus too, as the effects of exercise on blood glucose can last for up to 24 hours.

Pumps

Insulin pumps are programmable devices that automatically infuse insulin under the skin 24 h a day **(Fig. 5.2)**. All pumps deliver insulin through an infusion set—a tube that carries the insulin to a cannula (a small flexible tube) that's inserted under the skin. One pump has a very short cannula and sits on the skin, stuck down by adhesive, giving insulin through the very short tube. This pump stays on the body constantly. Most other types of pumps have longer tubing systems, which means that the pump can be disconnected from the body for some period of time. For

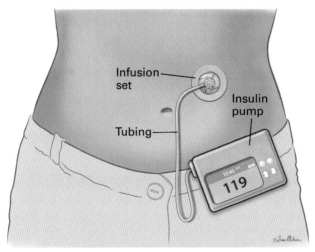

FIGURE 5.2   Insulin pumps contain enough insulin for several days. An infusion set carries insulin from the pump to the body through flexible plastic tubing and a soft tube or needle inserted under the skin.

both types of pumps, the cannula is inserted with a needle, which is then removed, leaving the cannula behind. The infusion set is changed every 2–3 days.

The pump is programmed by the user and health-care provider to deliver a basal rate, which is like long-acting insulin. It is a trickle of insulin delivered continuously as tiny mini-boluses. A person can have one or many basal rates depending on what their body needs. If a person's blood glucose level goes too low or they are going to do something like exercise, the pump can be turned off and the basal rate stopped.

One variable that the insulin pumps differ on is how low the basal rate can go. Some pumps can deliver as little as 0.025 units every hour and some can deliver as little as 0.05 or 0.1 units per hour. Infants or children with low insulin requirements may not be able to be on a pump that can only deliver the larger amount because it will be too much insulin for their body.

> Pumps require that the user input the blood glucose level and the amount of carbohydrate that is being eaten in order to give the bolus, or premeal, dose.

In addition, the pump is programmed to give bolus doses, which means that it can give a correction dose (to lower the blood glucose level if it is too high) and mealtime or carbohydrate doses, for food. The pump wearer must enter the carb content of the food and blood glucose level into the pump and tell the pump what to do—the pump only makes suggestions as to doses. The user has to decide in most cases. However, there is one pump that will stop giving insulin if the blood glucose level goes too low, and there is evidence that this low-glucose suspend feature reduces hypoglycemia. Pumps and sensors are increasingly beginning to work together to manage blood glucose levels independently. But currently most pumps require that the user input the blood glucose level and the amount of carbohydrate that is being eaten in order to give the bolus, or premeal, dose. The basal rate, however, is the insulin that marches through in a steady fashion and is stopped or adjusted only if the pump user decides to do so, as with most pumps. The basal rate may be automatically changed by certain pumps to help when the blood glucose levels goes too high or too low. These systems are called hybrid closed-loop systems.

Who Should Use a Pump?

Insulin pumps have been used successfully across the age spectrum. Whether to use a pump is a personal decision. People can manage their diabetes equally well with pumps or multiple injections, but some people prefer one method to another. This is not a lifelong commitment. Some people go on and off their pumps (but this should always be done with instructions from a person's diabetes team). Remember that a pump is just a tool—a person can reach blood glucose goals with a pump or injections. But here are some pros and cons to think about.

The one absolute requirement for using a pump is that the user and/or the user's caregivers are ready and willing to safely use the pump. This means that all of the tasks related to using a pump safely—and there are many—must be mastered and the person/family using the pump is capable of using it effectively. Most diabetes providers and insurance companies recommend or require that the person with type 1 diabetes check their blood glucose at least four times per day before they go on an insulin pump. If the pump stops working right, or the infusion set stops working, even for a few hours, the person using it can go into DKA (see Chapter 7), which is very serious and needs to be avoided. Checking blood glucose levels frequently will alert you to this possibility and will prevent the development of ketones.

People who might want to consider a pump include:

1. People who like the idea of a pump. If this is what the patient/parent wants, and they can use it safely, then it should be used.
2. Active people who benefit from changes in basal rates or suspending the pump when exercising.
3. People who have frequent low blood glucose reactions.
4. Anyone who has delays in the absorption of food from the stomach (gastroparesis).
5. Women planning pregnancy.
6. People who like the bolus calculator functions, including active insulin, that make it easier to determine insulin doses.

Downsides to an insulin pump include:

1. At present, an insulin pump doesn't take away the need to know premeal blood glucose levels and give insulin before meals.
2. There are technical aspects to using a pump—setting it up, putting it in, interacting with it—that are more complicated in some ways than using injections.
3. It only gives shorter-acting insulin. If it breaks or falls off, the person wearing it needs to be ready to give insulin by injection anywhere and at any time it is needed.
4. It is expensive, so find out which pumps are covered by your insurance.
5. All pumps are an extra piece of hardware attached to your body, either with tubing or attached to your skin. There are many clever ways to wear pumps, and hide them from view, but they do take a bit of getting used to at first.

Troubleshooting
The key to committing to a pump is to understand that troubleshooting is a constant requirement. Because the pump is giving you only rapid-acting insulin, if something happens and you don't get the insulin you think you/your child is supposed to be getting, blood glucose levels can go dangerously high. So high, in fact, that DKA can occur. Unfortunately pumps don't always alarm you when there is a small plug or clog in the infusion set or cannula. Sometimes the

tubing becomes loose and insulin drips outside of your body instead of under your skin. It is amazing all the ways in which getting insulin into the body can be messed up.

Be sure to check your blood glucose levels often enough to know if there is a problem. For most people this means checking ≥4–6 times per day at ~4-h intervals—before meals and bedtime and in the middle of the morning and afternoon.

If there is an explained high blood glucose level (and this number varies depending on the person), a correction dose should be given through the pump. Blood glucose should be measured again in 1–2 h. If the blood glucose level isn't going down as expected, the pump infusion set should be changed. Also, an injection of insulin should be given to be sure the insulin gets into your body. But this should be discussed with your health-care provider. Stay on top of these high blood glucose levels and pursue them until they come back down.

Testing for urine or blood ketones can be helpful to see how serious the problem is. If ketones are elevated, you should give insulin by injection, and you may need to contact your health-care provider. Be sure you work out a plan about how and when to ask for help.

> If ketones are elevated you may need to contact your health-care provider.

Return to Shotsville

"I was walking down a very crowded hall in the humanities building at the University of Tennessee when the wiring in my pump got caught in a door handle and flung off my body. An innocent bystander, hipster-type student, caught it (all University of Tennessee students are known for their football capabilities whether they play for the team or not). So, here we are in the middle of a busy building on a huge campus of over 27,000 students…. Me, tethered to my new best friend, and the hipster, who is basically holding my life in his hands. He said, "Cool beeper." I said, "Uh, that's a pump with my medication." He immediately throws the device back at me as if it were on fire. Apparently he wasn't comfortable with holding my lifeline (and I hope for the sake of us all he doesn't end up practicing medicine). Luckily I caught the pump and went on a mini vacation to what I called Shotsville.

Shotsville is great. Being pump-free and untethered made me feel like I owned my body again. That small, vestigial appendage was a source of irritation even if the irritation was more social than physiological. And, really, that's what I think management with type 1 diabetes has to include: the social ailments. This problem may not be huge but it is legitimate. So, I went on a pump break and then back on to the pump. I have had little difference in A1C and enjoy having the flexibility of therapy and, more importantly, the choice."

—Andy Rogers, 28, is pursuing his M.S. in physician assistant studies at Mercer University.

It's a Choice

Most people use their pump continuously, but it is not a permanent part of the body. Some kids use it during the school year but not during the summer. Others revert to injections when they go on vacation. Some have issues with their infusion sites, so they go off the pump for a while to let their sites recover. Whatever works to make diabetes treatment easier and better.

There are a number of pumps on the market; research what is best for you/ your child. Look at the individual pump company sites and read bloggers who have experience using the pumps. Speak with your diabetes team. Most insurance companies will not pay for a new pump more often than every 4 years, so this is a device you will have for a while. Finally, remember this is not a permanent decision. You can get a pump, wear it, stop wearing it, restart it— whatever works for you. It is an option for treating your diabetes and the choice is yours.

Beyond Insulin

The medications described in the sections that follow are not typically used by people with type 1 diabetes. Certain people may find them helpful.

Pramlintide

Besides insulin, the only other medication for type 1 diabetes that has been cleared by the FDA is pramlintide. This medication mimics another hormone in the body, called amylin, which, like insulin, is released from the β-cells. Because their β-cells are destroyed, people with type 1 diabetes are amylin-deficient. Pramlintide may help improve blood glucose levels and control body weight by slowing gastric emptying, suppressing glucagon production, and promoting satiety. However, it is a separate injection that must be given before meals whenever insulin is given. So it can be an added burden, even though it makes sense to give this hormone back along with insulin. It is not approved for people aged <18 years.

Metformin

Metformin is a medication that has been used for >50 years for the treatment of type 2 diabetes. It has potential benefits, which include positively affecting the heart, improving polycystic ovarian syndrome, and reducing the risk of cancer and possibly dementia. It has been used for the treatment of type 2 diabetes and prediabetes and is being studied as an anti-aging medication in people with normal glucose tolerance.

The side effects of metformin are well known and are generally related to the gastrointestinal system, including diarrhea, constipation, nausea, bloating, and vomiting. Many of the side effects of metformin can be reduced by starting with a low dose and going up slowly. Taking it with food and using the extended release form also helps. It also depletes the body of vitamin B12, so a supplement should be taken daily—the type that absorbs under the tongue.

Studies in people with type 1 diabetes have not shown much benefit in terms of A1C reduction. What it tends to do is to reduce the total daily insulin dose and may slightly aid in weight loss. In a study in adolescents with type 1 diabetes, metformin lowered the A1C and helped reduce the daily insulin dose and weight; however, it also increased the risk of severe low blood glucose reactions.

Children: Metformin is approved for the treatment of type 2 diabetes in both children and adults. It is not approved for the treatment of type 1 diabetes. However, in individual cases, along with the advice of your diabetes care team, its use can be considered. Generally this would be in an adolescent who is overweight and on higher doses of insulin who (if female) may also have polycystic ovarian syndrome. When starting metformin, insulin doses may need to be lowered in order to avoid low blood glucose reactions.

Adults: Metformin is the most commonly used medication for the treatment of type 2 diabetes. Because of its many potential benefits, adults with type 1 diabetes might want to consider using it off-label (meaning it is not approved for this use by the FDA) under the supervision of their health-care team. The reasons for using it include the presence of metabolic syndrome as well as polycystic ovarian syndrome (if female). Metabolic syndrome puts people at a higher risk of heart disease and stroke. It consists of central weight gain, insulin resistance (requiring more insulin than others to keep blood glucose levels in the normal range, which is usually >1 unit per kg per day), high blood pressure, and abnormal cholesterol levels (high triglyceride levels with low HDL cholesterol levels). Insulin-dose requirements often go down when metformin is added. In women who have had irregular periods, their menstrual cycles can become normal again, which is good, but it also can restore fertility, which may not be good unless pregnancy is desired.

GLP-1 RA

GLP-1 RA is a class of injectable medications that is used in people with type 2 diabetes that helps with blood glucose levels and weight loss. It mimics a normally occurring hormone known as GLP-1, which is a gut hormone. When people eat, this hormone is released. It helps insulin secretion occur more normally (not a benefit in type 1 diabetes unless a patient still makes some insulin), reduces glucagon levels, slows the emptying of the stomach, and makes people feel full.

In studies of people with type 1 diabetes, there has only been a slight benefit from using a GLP-1 RA. There is a high degree of individual variation in terms of response. The most common side effects are nausea, vomiting, and diarrhea. It should not be used in people who have had pancreatitis or medullary carcinoma of the thyroid.

Children: This class of medication is not approved for use in children with any type of diabetes and should be avoided until more information is available.

Adults: Some adult patients, particularly those with more slowly evolving type 1 diabetes, might already be taking a GLP-1 RA. If you and your diabetes health-care team decide that there is a benefit to taking the medication, then it could be continued. In someone with already diagnosed type 1 diabetes, it can be added, although it is an off-label use. A low dose should be started and gradually increased. A reduction in insulin dose may be needed, so be sure to monitor blood glucose levels and treat lows as needed. These agents may make you feel fuller and eat less, so less premeal insulin would be needed.

SGLT-2 Inhibitors

SGLT-2 inhibitors are a class of oral medications that lower blood glucose levels by increasing how much glucose is lost in the urine. The glucose is eliminated from the body, so there is less glucose in the blood. Along with this comes some weight loss and a decrease in the variability in blood glucose levels. This medication works well in both people with type 1 and type 2 diabetes but is only approved for use in people with type 2 diabetes. A big issue with this medication for people with type 1 diabetes is that it increases the risk of DKA, which is a serious problem. DKA can develop at normal blood glucose levels, which sometimes makes it hard to recognize. A similar medication that is an SGLT-1,2 inhibitor is being studied for people with type 1 diabetes, but also seems to have a low risk for DKA associated with it.

Children: No data are available for children, and given the risk of DKA, these medications should not be used in children outside of a clinical research study.

Adults: Some adults with type 1 diabetes have benefited from adding an SGLT-2 inhibitor to their insulin treatment. However, no matter how long someone has had diabetes, there is a higher risk of DKA when using these drugs. Therefore, unless your diabetes team members are very used to using this type of medication, it is not recommended. Should you and your team decide that you should use an SGLT-2 inhibitor, you must test your ketones (and know what the results mean), take only the lowest possible dose of the medication, and stop it if you get sick, dehydrated, have unexplained high blood glucose levels, or start a low-carbohydrate diet. A slight decrease in the dose of insulin may be needed when starting one of these medications, but the amount of carbohydrate eaten should stay the same.

Supplement Safety

Some people claim that certain supplements have magical blood glucose–lowering benefits—hello cinnamon—but the evidence is mixed at best. Supplements should never take the place of your diabetes medication, and the only proven benefits are for those who have documented deficiencies. Make sure to discuss any supplement use with your health-care providers.

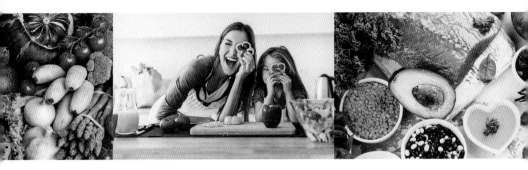

CHAPTER 6

Nutrition

In the past, being diagnosed with type 1 diabetes meant that one's diet had to change so that it fit the insulin regimen. Now it is the opposite—we try to create an insulin program to allow people to eat what they want, when they want to.

> There are a few key themes to a healthy diet: lots of fruits and veggies, plenty of whole grains and fiber, and limits on certain proteins, added sugars, and solid fats.

There is no "diabetes diet." What you eat can be based on your personal preferences, culture, traditions, and ethnicity in addition to your health goals. There are a few key themes to a healthy diet: lots of fruits and veggies, plenty of whole grains and fiber, and limits on certain proteins, added sugars, and solid fats.

It takes trial and error to understand the interplay between insulin dosing and various foods, and key to this process is to work with a registered dietitian (RD). Most people learn quickly as to what does and doesn't make blood glucose levels spike. For many people with type 1 diabetes (both young and old) this may mean learning a healthier way of eating, possibly eating less junk food and more vegetables, which is, frankly, the way everyone should be eating.

THE GOALS OF GOOD EATING

The American Diabetes Association has laid out the following goals of eating for health:

1. Attain and maintain:
   - Optimal blood glucose levels
   - Blood-fat levels that lower risk of heart disease
   - Blood pressure levels that lower risk of heart and kidney disease
2. Prevent and treat diabetes complications.
3. Fulfill personal nutritional needs, taking into account personal preferences and cultural food preferences. Mexican, Chinese, Greek, or whatever cuisine you prefer can be included in a healthy type 1 diabetes menu.
4. Keep the pleasure of eating by limiting foods ONLY when indicated by scientific evidence (or personal experience).

Each person with type 1 diabetes should work with a provider—ideally a registered dietitian who has expertise in type 1 diabetes—to establish an appropriate eating plan. This will include a strategy for synchronizing food, insulin doses, and physical activity. The overall strategy may change over time. Overweight and obesity can also be addressed in an eating plan.

FOUR KEY BEHAVIORS

The Diabetes Control and Complications Trial (DCCT), while not focused on nutrition, did identify four key behaviors associated with achieving a better A1C level.

1. Finding the right timing of meals and snacks that works in the person's life and adjusting that when life changes.
2. Adjusting insulin dose to match the meal size.
3. Treating high blood glucose levels promptly with insulin.
4. Avoiding the treatment of blood glucose lows with more carbohydrate than necessary.

Several other studies have found lower A1C levels in people who took a course on matching insulin doses to the carbohydrate content of food. What does such a course look like? Nutrition classes led by a registered dietitian, 3 or 4 sessions, each lasting 45–90 min, taken within 3–6 months of diagnosis. After that, an annual refresher is recommended.

If you're not able to go for a series of appointments, see a registered dietitian at least once so you can get a personalized meal plan. Ask your dietitian which online tools are good for reinforcing carbohydrate counting and assisting with keeping food records. For those smartphone-savvy folks, you can easily scan a favorite treat and a nutrition label will emerge. It's important that we all take advantage of the knowledge provided right at our fingertips, literally and figuratively.

NUTRITIONAL NEEDS THROUGH THE LIFE SPAN

Children and Adolescents

Your child's dietary requirements are no different from a child without diabetes. Focus on balanced and healthy eating. A great start is using the U.S. Department of Agriculture Choose My Plate guide for eating and adjusting it based on your child's preferences **(Fig. 6.1)**.

> A registered dietitian with experience in pediatric type 1 diabetes is a key member of the diabetes care team.

Another source for reliable nutrition and portion size information is the American Diabetes Association's Create Your Plate website (http://www.diabetes.org/food-and-fitness/food/planning-meals/create-your-plate), where you can create a variety of nutritious meals. See **Fig. 6.2** for an example of a nutritious meal.

It is difficult for a child with type 1 diabetes to watch siblings and parents eat whatever they want. Since family members without type 1 diabetes should be eating the same healthy well-rounded diet as the child with diabetes, it often helps to have the same food rules for the entire household. If the cookies aren't healthy for the child with diabetes, then the cookies are not healthy for the sibling without diabetes.

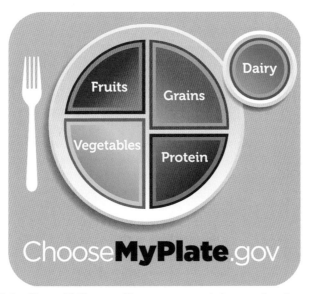

FIGURE 6.1   ChooseMyPlate.gov. These recommendations are for all ages.
Source: U.S. Department of Agriculture.

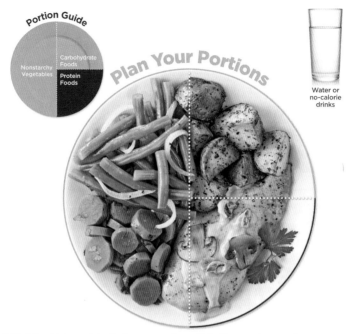

FIGURE 6.2 Using a 9-inch-diameter plate, fill half your plate with a variety of nonstarchy vegetables, a quarter of your plate with a carbohydrate food, and the remaining quarter with a low-fat protein-rich food.

You'll want to learn carbohydrate counting and how fiber, fats, and sugar alcohols may also affect your child's blood glucose levels. A registered dietitian with experience in pediatric type 1 diabetes is a key member of the diabetes care team. Your child's RD will help you devise—and revise as your child grows—a nutrition plan.

Most dread the initial visit with the CDE: "Oh no, I won't be able to eat my favorite chocolate bar!" or "My child won't be able to eat pizza like the rest of the kids at the birthday party!" All of those are just myths. Your child can still have pizza and chocolate. Meal plans are no longer as strict as they once were. These individualized meal plans will help you manage the amount of carbohydrates in each meal while still offering your child a balanced selection of food.

It's a good idea to start nutrition education at diagnosis and continue to get refreshers for at least that first year or so to cement the basic concepts. Then meet at least once a year with a registered dietitian to brush up skills, check that growth is on target, and reevaluate the meal plan. At times, you and your child may need more frequent visits to address rapid growth, nutritional needs that are in flux, and to transition the nutrition knowledge gradually from you to your child.

To determine the total amount of carbohydrates in the food your child eats, read food labels, which provide the total grams of carbohydrates per serving size. Making your famous grilled cheese and tomato soup for lunch at home? Going out for dinner? No worries, your dietitian will provide you the resources that contain the carbohydrate count of common foods as well as easily accessible online carbohydrate-counting tools.

It is helpful to eat consistent meals and schedule insulin injections at the same time every day. This helps prevent blood glucose levels from getting out of goal range. This aspect of type 1 diabetes management is challenging at certain ages. Teens are busier with social and after-school activities, and they are also transitioning to managing their diabetes without the help of their parents or caregivers. Toddlers tend to be grazers and getting them to sit down for scheduled meals/snacks can be challenging.

Weight

Childhood is a time of explosive growth, with caloric needs to match. Before diagnosis, type 1 diabetes can lead to weight loss, which needs to be restored after diagnosis by taking insulin, drinking fluids, and ensuring a healthy well-balanced diet.

> Insulin needs change as a child grows and develops, which can make it tricky.

Many believe that people living with type 1 diabetes tend to be lean. However, children living with type 1 diabetes are just as likely to be overweight and obese as children without diabetes.

Insulin needs change as a child grows and develops, which can make dosing insulin tricky. Too little insulin leads to weight loss and out-of-target blood glucose levels, while too much insulin can add extra pounds to a child's frame and results in frequent episodes of low blood glucose. Celiac disease and hyperthyroidism can also restrict weight gain, so if your child is underweight, screening for autoimmune diseases may be warranted. Track height, weight, and BMI throughout childhood, and check these values against what is healthy for a particular age.

Young Adults

Often there is a transition in dietary habits when a young person moves away from home for the first time. Away from the careful cooking of a concerned parent, the options for eating in college are often less healthy and unscheduled. For people with type 1 diabetes this can be a challenge, and this is a good time to see a registered dietitian to review how to approach the new food environment.

After high school or college, you might settle down into a more "routine" existence, perhaps living with a partner or roommates or living alone. Nutritional needs vary depending on your level of physical activity. If you are training for a marathon, you will need a different nutritional program than if you are a weekend warrior, playing basketball with your friends on the weekends. It's helpful to work with a dietitian to learn how to eat before, during, and after activity.

If you are in a serious relationship, consider bringing your significant other to a meeting with your dietitian. Food is an integral part of daily life, and it can help to have everyone understand its role in diabetes management. This doesn't mean that a spouse or partner should police your eating habits. Learning how to eat well together is the goal.

For women with type 1 diabetes, pregnancy is a unique challenge **(see p. 150)** and it should include nutritional advice from a qualified provider.

Adults

As we age, our basic metabolic rate falls and the number of calories we need to eat declines. People often say, "I don't understand why I'm gaining weight—I'm eating the same amount of food I always ate." And that is the answer—you can't eat the same amount of food you always ate and stay lean; you must gradually cut back your intake over time. This is true whether or not you have diabetes.

Diabetes may bring extra challenges. Complications such as gastroparesis, or heart or kidney disease, require dietary modification.

Even if you have no significant complications, visiting a dietitian for a refresher from time to time will be helpful, especially if your weight has changed.

Blueberries and Bagels

"At work, food is brought in for sharing, like birthday cakes, bagels, and homemade cookies. I'm the outlier who usually stays away from this type of food. My coworkers know I have type 1, they know I don't eat this food, and they respect me for it. They will also bring in fresh food like tomatoes, strawberries, and blueberries, sometimes from their backyards. When they bring in these foods, I join in. Some of them tell me, 'You know, I would be healthier if I ate like you.'

It is not easy to exercise self-control without the help of others. I'm fortunate that I have the support of those close to me. My wife and children appreciate the attention I pay to what I eat and when I eat. My wife does a lot of cooking, and when I tell her that a meal made me go high, we talk about it and plan so we can do better next time."

—Peter Madden

AN INSIDER'S GUIDE TO THE NUTRIENTS

Carbohydrates

Carbohydrates are one of three main nutrients found in food. (The other two are fat and protein.)

Foods with carbs include:

- Grains (cereal, bread, pasta, rice)
- Fruits and fruit juices
- Milk and yogurt
- Starchy vegetables and legumes (corn, peas, potatoes, and beans)
- Sweets
- Regular soft drinks and other sweetened beverages

When carbs are digested, they are converted into glucose, which enters the bloodstream. Even though carbs raise your blood glucose levels, foods with carbs are not "bad" and should not be avoided. Carbs provide you with energy and contain important minerals and vitamins. It is very important to eat enough carbs because they are used by the brain for energy. There are general guidelines as to how many carbs a person should eat that depend on age, weight, and physical activity.

Carbohydrate Counting

Keeping tabs on how much carbohydrate you/your child eats is a vital part of meal planning in type 1 diabetes. To help keep your blood glucose levels in your target range, your meal plan gives you a goal for how much carbohydrates to consume at meals and snacks. Some individuals are given a carbohydrate amount to eat with a set dose of insulin to match. Others are given a range of carbohydrate amount and an insulin-to-carbohydrate ratio to figure out the amount of insulin to give to match the amount of carbohydrates they plan to eat.

For a very simple example, let's assume a person's carb ratio is 1:15. This means the person takes 1 unit of rapid-acting insulin for every 15 g of carbs he eats. When he eats a piece of bread that has 15 g of carbs in it, he takes 1 unit of insulin. But when he eats a sandwich with two pieces of bread, then he is eating 30 g of carbs and thus takes 2 units. And if he adds a small apple, which is another 15 g of carbs, then he is eating 45 g of carbs, which requires 3 units of insulin. This is just an example. Your insulin-to-carb ratio might be different.

> Do the math based on the carb ratio that has been calculated by your diabetes team.

Clearly this takes practice. If you have an insulin pump, you can enter your carbs into the pump and it will do the math based on the carb ratio that has been calculated by your diabetes team. Sometimes you won't know exactly how much you will eat in advance, so it is okay to give some insulin before the meal and then another dose if more carbohydrates are eaten.

It is the total carb count that counts, but there are subtleties in terms of how different carbs affect your blood glucose level. This is why it is so important to meet with a dietitian to learn the basics of what works best for you. With your dietitian, you will figure out how to dose insulin for the carbohydrates eaten.

It is beyond the scope of this book to teach carbohydrate counting, and there are many resources to help you. It is a skill that requires some effort to learn at first. It will become second nature later.

Carbohydrate counting is easiest when at home, where portion sizes and food content can be controlled.

Sweets

Many people used to think that sugars, such as table sugar (sucrose), caused a more rapid and severe spike in blood glucose levels than starches. People with type 1 diabetes were told not to eat sweets. However, research studies have shown that gram for gram, sucrose and starch cause similar blood glucose responses in people with type 1 diabetes when given in the context of a meal with an identical composition of fat and protein.

But the situation is more complex than it seems at first. Eating carbohydrates alone, such as from a piece of hard candy, can quickly raise the blood glucose level and is used for treating low blood glucose reactions. But if you eat the same amount of sugar as a bowl of ice cream, which contains fat and protein, the blood glucose rise can be blunted. So the company a carbohydrate keeps affects how quickly the blood glucose level will rise.

Overall, we believe that for a given amount of insulin, carbs can be substituted for each other in a meal plan. This doesn't mean it's good to have sugary cereal for dinner and a candy bar for dessert. A diet with high levels of added sugar—sweeteners that are added to foods during processing—isn't going to be healthy, limiting essential nutrients and bumping up excess calories. It isn't good for anyone, diabetes or not.

Never Called It a Diet

"It's never been easy for me to lose weight. Ever. Once I reached my mid-30s, however, it became even more difficult. I would maintain my weight through activity—walking, swimming, Zumba—but maintenance was it.

A few years ago, my neighbors got together and formed a 'clean-eating' challenge for 30 days. I joined for the community, support, and accountability. In preparation for clean eating (loosely translated to all unprocessed foods), we shopped, read, and learned new recipes. And after a week, my family was hooked. We felt better, had more energy, and really enjoyed the recipes we were putting together. I even came across a recipe for pancakes that we could enjoy. I would make a batch and put them in the fridge for the week's breakfast. Even my then-6-year-old liked them! Thirty days came and went and we continued.

And one day, I stepped on the scale, and I had lost 25 pounds! And I was still motivated. I continued my daily activities of Zumba and walking and swimming in the summer. When I visited my endocrinologist, my A1C was lower and my daily insulin intake was reduced by 30%.

Since then, I have returned to eating some processed foods and drinking diet soda, but I do so in moderation. I find that I feel my best when I am eating unprocessed foods and can easily switch back and forth in my meals.

And I have maintained my weight loss. I'm very proud of that. I don't have a perfect body, and more than likely, I never will, but it's perfect for me. My blood sugar stays in range (most of the time) and that's my ultimate goal when it comes to diabetes management. I am adaptable to the changing needs of diabetes, especially when it comes to nutrition and weight maintenance.

The most interesting aspect of my experiment with clean eating is that I never called it a diet. It's not. It's a way of eating that works well for me with positive results in blood sugar management, weight maintenance, and a happy family. We continue to experiment with different grains and vegetables and create our own recipes with our favorite foods. Like diabetes, it's an ever-changing process."

—Anna Norton is CEO of DiabetesSisters, which creates programs and services to educate and support women living with diabetes.

Fiber and Whole Grain

Fiber is important to any diet. Fiber is found in vegetables, fruits, beans, and whole grains.

Fiber in food will slow the absorption of carbohydrates. But it is also considered a carbohydrate. So there needs to be some accommodation made for this when eating fiber-rich food. The general rule of thumb is that if food contains ≥5 g of dietary fiber per serving, subtract half the grams of dietary fiber from the total grams of carbohydrates (you can easily find this information on the Nutrition Facts label on packaged foods). The total equals the amount of carbohydrates you should use when calculating insulin requirements. For example, if food contains 12 g of carbohydrates and 6 g of fiber, the amount of carbs that will affect your blood sugar is 9 g.

Sugar Alcohols

Many people consume products made with sugar alcohols to manage calorie and sugar intake. Unlike regular sugar, sugar alcohols don't need insulin to be metabolized and won't cause a rise in blood glucose levels when consumed in controlled amounts. But if eaten in excess, these products will raise blood glucose levels and may cause gastrointestinal distress or other side effects. Talk with your diabetes team about achieving a reasonable nutritional balance.

Glycemic Index/Load

The glycemic index (GI) is a term that some people use to try and understand how much a given carbohydrate will raise the blood glucose level. Although this sounds complicated, it originated as a simple experiment: take 10 research subjects and feed them 50 g of carbohydrates from all sorts of different foods, such as table sugar, bread, fruits, corn, and carrots. Measure how high the blood glucose levels go after eating each single food and create a scale for ranking the response. The highest response (the food that raises the blood glucose the most) is 100, and foods that are in the range of ≥70 are called high-GI foods. These include glucose, white bread, high-fructose corn syrup, corn flakes, puffed rice, mashed potatoes, bagels, and waffles. Those in the range of 56–69 are medium-GI foods such as basmati rice, couscous, raisins, and cranberry juice. Those in the low-GI range of ≤55 raise the blood glucose levels the least and include legumes, fruits, starchy vegetables, and whole grains.

There are many factors that can affect the GI levels of these foods: ripeness and storage time (the riper the fruit or vegetable the higher GI level), processing (juice has a higher GI than whole fruit; mashed potato higher than baked), cooking method (how long food is cooked), and variety (brown rice vs. white rice). Think of an apple. If you drink apple juice, your blood glucose level goes up quite quickly; if you consume applesauce, your blood glucose level goes up a little more slowly; and if you eat an apple, intact fiber and all, your blood glucose goes up least of all.

The numbers associated with the GI are not really necessary to learn in order to count carbohydrates. However, the concept that some carbs increase the blood glucose levels more than others is a good one to know. And you will learn, by trial and error, what makes your blood glucose level go up the most and which the least.

Protein

Protein is an important part of the diet, and certain types of protein may be better for you than others. Over time, protein is turned into glucose in the body. If you eat a meal high in protein (which is often high in fat), you may need more insulin than the amount you calculate based on carb counting. In the beginning, however, it is best to consider protein fairly neutral in terms of the blood glucose rise. You can learn over time how to increase insulin for the protein content of the meal **(Table 6.1)**.

Fat

Fat may slow glucose metabolism or alter the timing of the glucose peak after a meal. It can slow gastric emptying and may increase insulin resistance. A higher-fat

TABLE 6.1   Proteins: Which to Eat, Which to Avoid

Often	Sometimes	Limit or avoid
Beef: top sirloin Extra lean ground beef, 96% lean, 4% fat	Beef: flank steak, strip steak, T-bone steak, filet mignon/tenderloin filet Lean ground beef: ≥93% lean, ≤7% fat	Beef: ribs, ground chuck, ribeye, porterhouse, sirloin steak Ground beef and ground beef patties: <93% lean, >7% fat
Eggs Cottage cheese: 0–1%	Reduced-fat cheese Cottage cheese: 2%	Cheese Cottage cheese: whole milk
Fish: salmon, tuna, mackerel, halibut, herring, sardines, trout, cod, catfish, anchovies	Lean deli meats: lean roast beef, turkey, or ham	Deli meats: roast beef, bologna, salami
Poultry: chicken and turkey without skin	Poultry: chicken and turkey with skin; chicken or turkey bacon/sausage	Processed meats: bacon, sausage, hot dogs, brats
Pork: pork loin, tenderloin, center loin	Pork: ham	Pork: ribs
Nuts: walnuts, almonds, peanuts/peanut butter, pecans, pistachios Legumes: beans, lentils, split peas Soy-based meat substitutes like tofu	Lamb	Untrimmed beef and pork

meal (e.g., ribs and brisket at your favorite BBQ joint) can affect postmeal blood glucose levels out of proportion to what you might anticipate based on the carbohydrates consumed. If you notice that your blood glucose levels rise after high-fat meals despite administering the appropriate amount of insulin, ask your diabetes health-care team about insulin adjustments. There are methods that can help address this issue based on your individual needs **(Table 6.2)**.

Alcohol can lower blood glucose levels.

Alcohol

Alcohol, in moderation, is fine for most people with diabetes—it may even be good for you—but the caveat is that alcohol can lower blood glucose levels. The American Diabetes Association recommends that men with diabetes limit their alcohol intake to no more than two drinks per day and women to no more than one per day. The body uses a special process to break down alcohol. That process takes away from the body's ability to make its own glucose from the liver (gluconeogenesis). So drinking alcohol can lower blood glucose levels afterwards, especially if consuming hard alcohol without a sweet mixer or dry wine or light beer.

Alcohol consumption can affect blood glucose levels for ≥24 h. It is very important to understand how your body and blood glucose levels react to the type of alcohol you drink—beer vs. wine vs. mixed drinks vs. shots. Do some trials at home in a safe environment before drinking in a social setting.

Usually it is recommended to avoid giving insulin for your first alcohol beverage and to check your blood glucose levels consistently during a night of alcohol consumption. Some people will need less insulin after drinking alcohol. It is a good rule of thumb to be sure to eat some carbohydrates along with drinking alcohol to help minimize the low blood glucose effect. If having a drink with a lot of sugar in it, such as fruit juice, you may need to take less

TABLE 6.2   Fats: Which to Eat, Which to Avoid

Often	Sometimes	Limit or avoid
Oils: canola, olive, sunflower, peanut	Oils: corn, soybean, safflower, sesame	Butter, lard, coconut oil
Trans-fat-free spreads	Mayonnaise	Margarine
Avocado, olives, seeds and peanut or almond butter.		Cream
Oil-based salad dressing: vinaigrette, oil & vinegar	Low-fat cream–based salad dressing: light Ranch	Full-fat cream–based salad dressing such as Ranch or blue cheese

All fats are high in calories, so keep the portion size small (<1 Tbsp in most cases).

insulin than anticipated for the juice carbohydrates. Discuss strategies for safe alcohol use with your health-care team.

Discuss alcohol use with your diabetes care teams. Avoid binge drinking. Be sure to drink with friends who are aware that you have type 1 diabetes. Being drunk and being hypoglycemic can sometimes look alike, and it is important not to confuse the two. If you begin to vomit after drinking, your friends should seek care at an emergency department to be sure you aren't in DKA (see Chapter 7).

In terms of calorie content, gram for gram alcohol is just a little less than fat. People using SGLT-2 inhibitors off-label should avoid excess alcohol.

Celiac Disease

In celiac disease, the immune system attacks the intestines but causes harm only in the presence of one food component: gluten. This protein bundle is found in wheat, barley, rye, and related grains. People with celiac disease need to meticulously avoid gluten both in foods as well as in medications and supplements. The FDA requires that foods labeled as gluten-free contain less than 20 parts per million of gluten, which may make them safe for people with celiac disease. Getting adequate nutrition, maintaining bone health, and keeping blood glucose on target can take a bit more practice and patience for people with celiac disease; an RD with expertise in type 1 diabetes and celiac disease is essential for learning how to live with dual diseases.

Low-Sodium Diet

If you have high blood pressure, a dietitian may recommend a low-sodium diet. To start on a low-sodium diet, the first step is not to add salt to your food. This means all table salt or sea salt. There are some salt substitutes, but your dietitian may advise against using them. Many contain extra potassium, which may not be safe if you are taking certain medications. Check with your pharmacist. Use herbs and spices for seasoning.

A major source of salt in the diet comes from packaged and prepared foods. Read food labels for salt content as well as the carbs. It is often surprising how much salt the food we regularly eat contains. The many apps that track caloric intake will also calculate salt intake, and they can teach you how close you are to your reduced-salt goal.

Renal Diet

Diet is one of the important treatments in managing diabetes and kidney disease. You will need to work with a registered dietitian to create an eating plan. This plan will help manage blood glucose levels and reduce the amount of waste and fluid your kidneys process. Your dietitian will give you nutritional guidelines on how much protein, fat, and carbohydrates as well as potassium, phosphorous, sodium, and fluids you can consume each day.

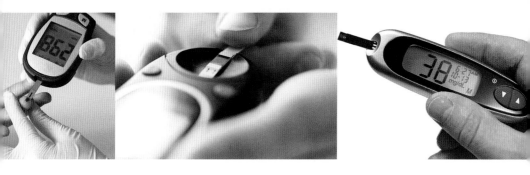

Chapter 7

Highs and Lows

HYPOGLYCEMIA

Rush and Fog

"There are the slow lows, where blood sugars drop ever so slightly over time until you are symptomatic. There are the crashing lows, where due to insulin or exercise (or both), I'm crashing down at a rapid pace and feel terrible. These are the ones that make me feel weak, shaky, nervous, not want to talk to anyone, and give me a ravenous need to eat everything around me until I feel better. It's like an adrenaline rush and brain fog mixed into one. I hate this feeling. My husband knows to leave me alone when I'm low (it's the only time I don't like to be touched or talked to), unless I ask for help. I do like that he will bring me a juice box or something to treat at night. It helps to have a little bit of the burden shared by someone else."

—Natalie H. Strand, MD, is a pain management specialist, a mother of two, and was a member of the first two-woman team to win *The Amazing Race.*

A blood glucose level that is too low is called hypoglycemia. "Hypo" means low, and glycemia refers to glucose levels. Experts typically define hypoglycemia as a blood glucose level of <70 mg/dL, while severe hypoglycemia is a loss of consciousness or inability to self-treat to raise blood glucose. Hypoglycemia is the limiting factor in achieving normal blood glucose and A1C levels. Consider hypoglycemia when setting blood glucose targets. Avoiding severe lows is more important than having an A1C of 6%.

You may wonder why people without diabetes don't usually have blood glucose lows. This is because they have two lines of defense against low blood glucose. When their blood glucose starts to fall, for example when exercising, their body makes less insulin and increases glucagon levels, which raises blood glucose. These adjustments are beautifully choreographed and keep blood glucose levels in balance.

These responses aren't available to people with type 1 diabetes. Their α-cells don't make glucagon normally in response to hypoglycemia. And once insulin is given via injection or pump, it can't be taken back or turned off like insulin made by a functioning pancreas.

> The symptoms of hypoglycemia are a good warning sign; being unaware of falling blood glucose levels can cause serious problems.

Symptoms

A low blood glucose level triggers the release of epinephrine (adrenaline), the "fight-or-flight" hormone. That's why a low can cause a thumping heart, sweating, tingling, and anxiety.

If the blood glucose level continues to drop, the brain does not get enough glucose and stops functioning as it should. This can lead to blurred vision, difficulty concentrating, confused thinking, slurred speech, numbness, and drowsiness. Prolonged starvation of the brain may lead to seizures, coma, and very rarely death.

Hypoglycemia Unawareness

Unpleasant as they may be, the symptoms of low blood glucose are useful. These symptoms tell you that you need to take swift action to bring your glucose levels back into a safe range.

Hypoglycemia Symptoms

Here are signs and symptoms of hypoglycemia—from milder, more common indicators to most severe. Signs are things others can notice, while symptoms are sensations that only the person with diabetes can notice and express.

Shakiness	Tingling or numbness in the lips or tongue
Nervousness or anxiety	
Sweating, chills, and clamminess	Headaches
Irritability or impatience	Weakness or fatigue
Confusion	Anger, sadness, or stubbornness
Rapid/fast heartbeat	Lack of coordination, clumsiness
Light-headedness or dizziness	Nightmares or crying out during sleep
Hunger and nausea	
Color draining from the skin (pallor)	Bizarre behavior
Sleepiness	Seizures
Blurred/impaired vision	Unconsciousness

However, some people don't get these early symptoms. If hypoglycemia occurs too frequently, the body gets used to hypoglycemia and stops sending out the adrenaline alert every time blood glucose dips too low. This is called hypoglycemia unawareness. The first symptoms are the ones that occur when the brain is not getting enough glucose.

Hypoglycemia unawareness puts the person at increased risk of severe low blood glucose reactions (when a person may pass out or have a seizure). People with hypoglycemia unawareness need to take extra care to check blood glucose frequently, particularly prior to and during critical tasks such as driving. A continuous glucose monitor can be a huge help, which can sound an alarm for a falling as well as a low blood glucose level.

It's possible to get your early symptoms back by careful avoidance of any, even mild, hypoglycemia for several weeks. This generally means increasing your target blood glucose level (a new target that needs to be worked out with your diabetes care team) and may even result in a high A1C level, but regaining the ability to sense lows is worth the temporary rise in blood glucose levels.

Clouded Bravery

"Many people say that I'm brave because I poke myself multiple times in a day with fingersticks or syringes. But many don't understand that the hardest, scariest, and most paralyzing moments have nothing to do with a needle.

Usually I notice it with a shift of my head. It will feel like things move slightly slower than they should. I'll mentally calculate, 'When did I last eat? How much insulin did I take?' And even though neither of these things matter because they could have nothing to do with my low blood sugar, I try to rationalize that I'm fine.

I can feel my heart beating out of my chest, and it becomes difficult to hear and see. Check blood sugar level, get sugar. Except I forgot to replace the sugar in my purse the last time I used it, so now I'm a fool without the one thing I need. I start rummaging through my purse, hoping for some random piece of candy, something, anything, that can bring my levels up. I can go get a soda from the machine, but I don't have any cash.

I need someone to help me, but in this intense moment of fear, my brain becomes incapacitated and all logical ideas are gone. Everything is so blurry, I can hardly make out what I'm even looking at now.

The only way to move past the fear is to robot-like move forward. Get up and go find something or someone to help. Saying to someone 'I have low blood sugar and need juice' becomes the hardest sentence I've ever said; shame overwhelms me and the effects of the low make it difficult for me to even move my mouth, let alone say something that makes sense. I'm going to die right here, all because I didn't put more emergency sugar in my purse. Because I'm a bad diabetic.

When I finally obtain the sugar I need, I can't turn off the panic coursing through my veins. I'll inhale the food and guzzle the soda quicker than I can even realize. Often I'll try to drink the soda again, confused why the bottle is empty. The world is still spinning for me, my heart still feels like it's beating so quickly that it'll explode. It can take me 30 minutes to convince myself that I'm not dying, that I have pulled through this again.

This experience never gets easier. Knowing that I've survived it a million times before doesn't help me believe I'll get through in again. After 16 years of this, I still struggle to hold back the tears and shame and to fight for myself in that moment. It all seems so simple: if it's an emergency, ask someone to help and very likely, they will. But it's hard to remember that when all you can identify is the sense of death being near.

Every diabetic has their story (or stories). The time they don't know how they even came through, how they wandered aimlessly and mute through a grocery store trying to figure out what to do but because they were so low they just couldn't make sense of anything. These are the moments that make us brave. These are the moments where we must have a stronger sense in us to live and fight for it than to let go and let the dizzying wheel take us away. These are the moments that no matter how much you love a diabetic, you will never truly understand.

Ours is a disease where you can do everything right all day, but then you might have to stare down death in the face and get up and move along as if everything is fine. Because it is. You lived. No one sees the chemical, hormonal, emotional scars. So brave, yes, but for so many reasons others may never understand."

—DeAnna Wendland, 33, teaches middle school history, English, and religion, and plans her road trips around craft beer and delicious wine.

Causes of Lows

Hypoglycemia is common; the average person with type 1 diabetes experiences an estimated two episodes of mild hypoglycemia each week, and that's only counting those episodes with symptoms. Adding in asymptomatic and overnight hypoglycemic events would likely drive that number up.

> Almost all lows have a cause, although sometimes it is hard to figure out exactly why they happened.

Insulin

Too much insulin is a sure route to hypoglycemia. One reason newer insulins are preferred over NPH and regular insulin is that they're less likely to cause blood glucose lows, particularly overnight. Insulin pumps may also reduce the risk of hypoglycemia. Accidentally injecting the wrong insulin type or an excessive dose of insulin or injecting directly into the muscle, instead of the subcutaneous tissue, can cause hypoglycemia.

Food

Eating foods with less carbohydrates than usual may lead to hypoglycemia if insulin isn't lowered to compensate. How much of your caloric intake comes from liquids versus solids can also affect blood glucose levels. Liquids are absorbed much faster than solids, so timing the insulin dose to the absorption of glucose from foods can be tricky. The composition of the meal—how much fat, protein, and fiber are present—can affect the absorption of carbohydrates.

Physical Activity

Exercise has many benefits. The tricky thing for people with type 1 diabetes is that it can lower blood glucose in both the short- and long-term. Nearly half of children in a type 1 diabetes study who exercised an hour during the day experienced a low blood glucose reaction overnight. The intensity, duration, and timing of exercise can all affect the risk of going low.

Treatment

For mild or moderate episodes of hypoglycemia—basically any time you can treat yourself—the "Rule of 15" applies.

Here's what to do when blood glucose dips to <70 mg/dL:

1. Consume 15 g of simple carbohydrates if blood glucose is 50–70 mg/dL. Up to 30 g if blood glucose is <50 mg/dL.
2. Wait 15 min.
3. Check blood glucose again.
4. If the level is still <70 mg/dL, repeat steps 1–3.
5. Repeat until blood glucose is >70 mg/dL and then consider eating a snack or small meal to keep levels from dropping again.

This stepwise approach can help you avoid overtreatment, which can lead to high blood glucose.

Children: Young children usually need <15 g to fix a low blood glucose level: infants may need 6 g, toddlers may need 8 g, and small children may need 10 g. This needs to be individualized for the patient, so discuss the amount needed with your diabetes team.

Good for Treating Lows*	Poor Choices for Treating Lows
Glucose tablets or gel	Ice cream, milkshake
Honey (not for age <1 year)	Donuts
Regular soft drinks	Pizza
Fruit juice	Candy bars
No- or low-fat milk	Nuts, cheese, meat
Raisins	Pies, cakes, cookies
Hard candies	Potatoes, French fries, chips

*Check the Nutrition Facts and know how much the "dose" should be for you or your child.

When treating a low, the choice of carbohydrate source is important. According to some research, people with a history of severe hypoglycemia tend to treat their lows with foods that don't raise blood glucose rapidly. Complex carbohydrates or foods that contain fats along with glucose can slow the absorption of glucose and should not be used to treat an emergency low.

Tips for Treating Low Blood Glucose

- If you are not able to check your blood glucose and you think it's low, treat the symptoms regardless. Low glucose can be dangerous if not treated, so it's better to be safe.
- Make sure to eat a mixed meal or snack after treating low blood glucose. This should consist of fat, protein, and carbs. It helps to prevent a fall in blood glucose once the simple carbs "wear off." Discuss how much insulin to give for this post-low-carb intake with your diabetes team. Some insulin is almost always needed to prevent a rebound high.
- When calculating your carbohydrate dose, do not count the carbs taken to treat low blood glucose.
- Do not overtreat a low. Eating or drinking too much carbs could cause your blood glucose levels to go too high.
- Record any low blood glucose levels in in your record book/electronic log, noting causes (exercise, too much insulin, not enough food) to discuss with your diabetes care team.
- Sometimes drinking water while waiting to recover from a low is helpful— the symptoms from a low blood glucose reaction may persist after the low has been treated. Drinking water can help satisfy the urge to have more carbs.

"Sometimes in the middle of an argument, my husband will say, 'Go test your sugars, Babe,' which you think would be really frustrating. Except, even when he's mad, he can tell when my blood sugars are low. Even when he's mad, he cares enough to stop being mad. Just long enough for me to drink 4 oz of juice though."

—Amirah Meghani

Sometimes, it feels safer to keep blood glucose levels higher, to avoid hypoglycemic episodes.

Severe Hypoglycemia

Severe hypoglycemia can cause a loss of consciousness, seizure, coma, or an inability to eat or drink fast-acting carbs to correct a low. This is the scenario that requires help from your family, friends, roommates, coworkers, or other people in your life. They'll need training to recognize severe hypoglycemia and to administer glucagon. Every person with type 1 diabetes should have a nonexpired glucagon kit somewhere nearby in case of emergency, but it also requires that someone else is capable of using it. If this isn't the case, then 911 should be called so that paramedics can treat the low blood glucose reaction. This is why it is helpful if people with type 1 diabetes carry some form of identification, so the need for immediate treatment with glucagon or intravenous glucose is easily understood. Ask your health-care team for information on forms of identification, from old-school bracelets to trendy dog tags. These should say "Type 1 Diabetes, Insulin."

Glucagon is a glucose-raising hormone, the anti-insulin. Glucagon kits contain the hormone in a powdered form that should be mixed with the saline included in the kit and injected under the skin as you would insulin or into the muscle. The dose of glucagon depends on age and body size. The recommendation is to inject 10–30 µg/kg body weight, or, if weight isn't known, 0.5 mg for people aged <12 years and 1.0 mg for those >12 years. The kits have detailed instructions and are meant to be used easily in the event of an emergency. It is good to ask your CDE or RN to review glucagon instructions yearly with family members and caregivers. This may prevent panic and uncertainty if and when dosing is needed. Don't throw away unused, expired kits—have family, friends, roommates, coaches, teachers, or school nurses practice mixing up expired glucagon kits and giving an injection to an orange. There are good online tutorials and apps on how to give a glucagon injection.

Hypoglycemia can trigger confusion and mental slowing during an event and may cause some long-term harm, particularly if severe low blood glucose reactions happen frequently. Episodes of severe and prolonged low blood glucose levels may cause subtle forms of brain damage, and there may be slight changes on cognitive tests. Overall, though, the effect of hypoglycemia on brain function is likely to be small and may depend on the age at which hypoglycemia occurs. As people age, these episodes tend to happen more often. This then becomes something of a vicious cycle because older brains in general tend toward cognitive decline.

Fear of hypoglycemia is common in adults and children with type 1 diabetes. Children with type 1 and their parents report the most fear. Vigilantly avoiding and treating lows is critical, certainly, but don't let fear get out of control. Talk to a provider if concerns about hypoglycemia become crippling.

Children: Infants and toddlers are at particular risk when they develop hypoglycemia because they can't understand and verbalize their symptoms. A study of children using continuous glucose monitors found that their blood glucose dipped to <50 mg/dL on 35% of nights, with durations of up to 2 h.

For children who are sick or unable to consume enough to raise blood glucose sufficiently, mini-doses of glucagon may be given to treat episodes of mild or moderate hypoglycemia. This means giving less than the full dose needed to bring someone back from a severe episode of hypoglycemia but enough to treat more mild events. It can prevent a mild low from becoming more serious in a child who won't eat. It also cuts the number of calories that need to be eaten to treat a low.

Here's how (and be sure to check with your diabetes team to be sure this is all right):

1. Mix glucagon per instructions.
2. Draw up glucagon from the vial in an insulin syringe INSTEAD of the syringe that comes with the kit. Dose in insulin syringe units is determined based on age:

    <2 years = 2 units on an insulin syringe
    ≥2–15 years = 1 unit on an insulin syringe per year of age
    >15 years = 15 units on an insulin syringe (maximum dose)
3. Give glucagon as you would insulin: under the skin, not in the muscle.
4. Measure blood glucose in 30 min and again in 1 h, then every hour after.
5. If in 30 min blood glucose is <100 mg/dL, you can give another dose of glucagon, but the dose should be doubled. Recheck blood glucose in 30 min. If glucose does not rise after the second dose and your child cannot take rapid-acting carbs by mouth, call your diabetes team. Your child may need to go to the hospital for intravenous fluids and glucose.
6. This sequence can be repeated every 2 h during an illness. The glucagon mixed in the vial can be used for up to 24 h. Remember to pick up another glucagon kit from the pharmacy so that you always have a backup. Make sure that your child is taking in carbohydrates in the form of liquids or solids so that their glucose stores in the muscles and liver are replenished. If they are unable to take in carbs during the illness, the glucose stores will be depleted and the glucagon won't work. In this case, your child may need to go to the hospital for intravenous hydration and glucose. If the glucagon needs to be repeated a second time, make sure to update your diabetes team and follow their recommendations.

Adults: Throughout adulthood, rates of hypoglycemia persist, with more frequent mild episodes and an ongoing risk of severe hypoglycemia. Older individuals have the highest rates of severe hypoglycemia and often develop hypoglycemia unawareness. Low blood glucose levels in older adults occur frequently, no matter what the A1C level, and older adults often have other disorders, such as heart disease, that make them more vulnerable to side effects caused by low blood glucose levels. Additionally, older people often live alone, without a partner or caregiver to help with the treatment of hypoglycemic events.

Caregivers: It can be very upsetting to see someone you care about develop a low blood glucose reaction and feel that there is nothing you can do. Fortunately, you are not powerless. These steps are often helpful:

1. If you observe behaviors that you recognize as associated with a low blood glucose reaction, you can gently ask if the person is having a low blood glucose reaction. Sometimes people become a bit belligerent when they are low, but a gentle suggestion can be helpful.

2. Offer to get some juice or other form of simple sugar to treat the low, and the person's meter. You CANNOT force someone to eat or drink if they don't want to do so, so don't try.

3. If the person is looking confused and losing the ability to think clearly, help them sit down or lie down. Be calming and continue to offer juice or other simple carbohydrates.

4. If a person becomes unconscious or has a seizure, make sure they are safely on the floor. Turn their head to the side so they don't choke on their saliva. Do not put your fingers in the person's mouth. Give a glucagon shot, if you have glucagon and know how to use it. If in doubt about what to do, call 911.

5. Remember, as long as you are there to help, the person is going to be fine. Even if the person is unconscious they will recover as soon as their blood glucose level comes back up. This can be frightening to observe, but it is not a heart attack or a stroke, just a lack of glucose in the brain.

6. After someone recovers from a low blood glucose reaction, particularly a severe low blood glucose reaction, they will need to eat a meal or a snack containing protein, fat, and carbohydrates. Otherwise a low blood glucose reaction could happen again.

Prevention of Lows

Monitoring blood glucose, with either a meter or a continuous glucose monitor, is the tried and true method for avoiding hypoglycemia. Studies consistently show that the more a person checks blood glucose, the lower his or her risk of hypoglycemia. Check before and after meals, before and after exercise (or during, if it's a long or intense session), and before bed. After intense exercise, also check in the middle of the night. Check more amidst change: a new insulin routine, a different work schedule, an increase in physical activity, or travel across time zones.

Data Dump

If hypoglycemia has you stumped, bring a record of blood glucose, insulin, exercise, and food data to a health-care provider, who can help sleuth out a cause of lows. The more information you give your health-care provider, the more they can help analyze your situation. Hypoglycemia may be prevented, for example, by adjusting the timing of insulin dosing, exercise, and meals or snacks. Changing insulin doses or the types of food consumed may also do the trick.

DKA

DKA is a severe life-threatening condition that means you have too many ketones in your body. Ketones are caused by the breakdown of fat when there isn't enough insulin to meet your body's needs. When they build up, the result is acidosis (too much acid in the blood). If not treated, this can lead to death. Usually blood glucose levels are elevated (>250 mg/dL) but not always. It is the presence of too many ketones in the blood and urine that defines DKA.

Her Face Went White

"I developed type 1 diabetes in 1974 when I was 18 and in my first year of college. I began having all of the classic symptoms but didn't know what that meant. I just knew I felt like hell. Working too hard, eating badly, and perhaps a bit sick, I thought. After about three weeks, I returned home for spring break. While having breakfast I told my mother I had been feeling poorly and couldn't see very well. She turned to me and said, 'Come here.' Huh? Why? But I got up and walked to her. She stepped up to my face and said, 'Breathe on me.' I was completely confused, but you don't argue with Mother. I blew out a breath, and her face went white. She was smelling for acetone, a sign of untreated diabetes. Her father was diabetic and she knew that smell from her child-hood. Within an hour I was admitted to the hospital."

—Sean McLin is a director of photography for motion pictures and television. He has had diabetes since 1974.

About one out of three children have DKA at diagnosis; the number isn't known in adults, but there are an estimated 130,000 cases (type 1 and type 2) of DKA in the U.S. every year. DKA is more common and frequently more severe in children diagnosed with type 1 diabetes aged <5 years, possibly due to delayed

---

Symptoms of DKA

Symptoms of DKA should not be ignored and should prompt a call to a provider or trip to the emergency department.

Early symptoms of diabetes ketoacidosis:
- Thirst or a very dry mouth
- Frequent urination
- High blood glucose levels (typically >250 mg/dL, although ketones can occur at lower levels)
- High levels of ketones in the urine or blood

Later symptoms of diabetes ketoacidosis:
- Constantly feeling tired
- Dry or flushed skin
- Nausea, vomiting, or abdominal pain
- Difficulty breathing, chest pain
- Fruity odor on the breath
- A hard time paying attention
- Confusion

diagnosis or because type 1 diabetes progression is more aggressive in younger ages. DKA is more common in people who have higher A1C levels and less common as people become older.

The Biology

While high blood glucose can be associated with DKA, hyperglycemia alone will not cause DKA. Insulin deficiency is at the root of DKA. Without insulin, cells can't absorb glucose from the bloodstream. The body interprets this as starvation and sets into motion a variety of emergency starvation-avoidance systems. For starters, the liver starts to break down its glucose stores, releasing them into the blood, worsening high blood glucose. At the same time, the liver starts cobbling together new molecules of glucose from bits and pieces of other nutrients in the body.

The main driver of DKA is the third anti-starvation protocol: burning fats and turning them into chemicals called ketone bodies that the body can use as fuel in place of glucose. The ketone bodies are acids and, as they accumulate in the body, can override the blood's buffering system, which normally maintains the pH within a narrow life-sustaining range. Ketones spill into the urine, and it's a good thing they do, because ketones act as an early warning system that can help prevent DKA.

> DKA can be caused by insulin lack as well as not giving enough insulin when sick or stressed. This can happen even with normal blood glucose levels.

Causes

Illness is a common precipitating factor in DKA because the body's response to sickness is to release hormones that can act to counter insulin, raising blood glucose. Also, because a person may not be able to eat, insulin doses at mealtime may not be taken, leading to insulin deficiency. A third factor is dehydration, which can come along with vomiting and inadequate fluid consumption. That's why it's critical to follow sick-day rules.

Insulin deficiency, and DKA, can also onset rapidly in the event of an insulin pump malfunction. Take note that a common cause of DKA in pump users is not using backup insulin (in pens or syringes) when blood glucose is high or ketones are detected in the urine.

Another unfortunate cause of DKA is insulin omission. Some people don't take insulin because they can't afford it, they don't know how to take the medication properly, or they have a fear of insulin. Other people purposefully skip insulin doses for weight management purposes, particularly adolescent girls. DKA is associated with a variety of psychosocial factors, including an unstable or dysfunctional family, language barriers, psychiatric or eating disorders, and financial insecurity. DKA is seen in people who have the highest A1C levels, especially in teenagers and transitioning adults, indicating that an overall lack of adherence with diabetes management can lead to serious acute issues.

Treatment of DKA

There are four main treatments: fluids, insulin, potassium, and treating the cause.

Fluids: High glucose spills into the urine, drawing out water and minerals and causing high urine output at the beginning. This, along with possible vomiting, contributes to dehydration. Unless a person is able to drink enough fluids on their own, giving fluids through an intravenous line will be needed. It treats the dehydration and stops the formation of ketones. In children, this is done very carefully—too much fluid given to treat DKA can be harmful. Adults are more tolerant of fluids and are generally given a fairly large amount ($\geq$1 L) initially to help them return to normal.

Insulin: At the same time the fluids are given, an intravenous line with insulin in it will be started. The insulin will be directly dripped into the vein so it can act quickly to turn off ketone production and restore the body to normal. In some cases giving frequent insulin injections also works. At the point of treating DKA, most people are in the emergency room of a hospital, so the hospital's protocol for treating DKA will be followed. Regardless, giving insulin by some route is vital for treating this condition.

Potassium: This vital electrolyte is often depleted in DKA. Even if starting levels are high or normal, the potassium levels can fall, and this is very serious because adequate potassium levels are required for a normal heartbeat. Potassium is given intravenously or orally, or both. When given through the vein, it can hurt a bit, but it is well worth it. Definitely needed in most cases of DKA.

Treating the cause: If there is an infection, such as a bladder infection or pneumonia, this needs to be treated. Older adults may be having a heart attack or other serious problem, so the team in the emergency room will need to carefully check out all the possible problems that can be happening at the same time.

Once treatment is started, a person starts to feel much better within a few hours. The vomiting and headache (caused by the ketones) stop, normal urine flow returns, and the person "comes back to life." It is different in a child where this could be the first signal that they have diabetes—the DKA means the beginning of learning to deal with insulin injections and life as a person with diabetes. But in a person who already has diabetes, usually within 12–24 h they are able to resume their normal insulin treatment plan and go home. In many cases if caught early, steps can be taken to avoid the entire event.

Children: Approximately one-third of children with new-onset type 1 diabetes are in DKA when they are diagnosed. DKA can also happen when children do not get enough insulin when they are sick with an illness, when their insulin pump stops working and the child or family does not realize that this is the cause of the high blood glucose levels, or when too many insulin doses are missed.

DKA at the diabetes diagnosis is overwhelming and scary for the child and the parents. The child may be in an ICU with more than one intravenous line attached to monitors that are beeping and getting frequent blood draws.

Parents often feel guilty that they didn't realize that something was wrong sooner and worry that they did something to have caused the diabetes. Both of these feelings are natural but are simply not true. Sometimes it is hard to recognize increased thirst and urination in kids because they are still in diapers, are at school using the water fountain and restroom on their own, or are teenagers and private about these matters. Even some health-care providers have a hard time recognizing symptoms of diabetes in a child and don't test for diabetes. If there is another family member with type 1 diabetes, children and adults can be screened for the antibodies in the blood that are associated with developing type 1 diabetes. If the antibodies are positive, then the family knows that they are at risk of developing type 1 diabetes and can be on the lookout for symptoms. Screening family members lowers the rate of DKA at diagnosis.

On Day 9

"On the day we began a cross-country move, our 15-month-old vomited all over the airport terminal. John threw up four more times over the next eight days. He was otherwise happy, despite waking up several times a night for bottles. We attributed that to the unfamiliar surroundings. After all, we did take him to the pediatrician after a few days and were told it was a virus.

On Day 9 of this 'virus,' John was lethargic and refusing to eat or drink. One finger prick at the emergency room and all the pieces fell into place. Our boy has type 1 diabetes and was in DKA. The next 48 hours in the PICU were the scariest we have ever experienced. Four more days of training with a team of educators and we were sent home with an insulin pump on our toddler.

While in the hospital, I feared that my happy, easygoing boy would never be the same, but John was playing with his sister within minutes of getting home. Six months later, we just returned from a family vacation full of airplanes, water parks, and even ice cream. Planning ahead, site changes, and BG checks are now routine. John is as happy as ever with a lifetime of possibilities ahead of him."

—Betsy Lennane

Adults: Often DKA in adults occurs either because of an illness that isn't treated properly with increased insulin doses and carbohydrates or because of a lack of access to medical care, which means patients can't get their insulin prescriptions refilled and run out of insulin. Unfortunately, the latter situation happens far too often in underserved regions of the U.S. and around the world. Sometimes young adults and sometimes older adults simply rebel and stop giving enough insulin. Adults with new-onset type 1 diabetes have DKA seemingly less often than children.

Adults (and children) with diabetes must NEVER run out of insulin. A pharmacy can give you regular insulin (a vial and syringe) without a prescription if you can prove you have diabetes. Generally you can prove this by bringing in an empty vial of insulin or a pen or your meter—something that shows you have diabetes. You can give a dose of regular insulin every 6 h and keep enough insulin in your body. You can also go to any urgent-care center or emergency room and tell them you have diabetes and need insulin. With type 1 diabetes, you often must fight to get what you need. But getting insulin is possible even when access to a diabetes doctor may not be.

Call your health-care team if:

- You need help determining your insulin dose.
- Your blood glucose levels are >250 mg/dL for >2 days.
- You have moderate or large ketones.
- You are not able to tolerate small sips of fluid.
- You child has diarrhea or has been vomiting for >6 h.

Insulin Guidelines for Sick Days

Type of Insulin	Insulin Guidelines
NPH and short-acting, or premixed insulin	• If you are able to eat and drink carbs, take your usual insulin dose. • If you are not able to eat or drink your usual amount of carbs AND your glucose levels are <250 mg/dL, reduce your usual insulin doses by 50%. • If you are not able to eat or drink carbs for an extended period of time, call your health-care provider for advice.
Background and mealtime insulin	• Always take your usual dose of background insulin. • Match your mealtime insulin dose to your carb intake. • If you have a correction factor, use it before meals if your blood glucose is >200 mg/dL. If you are not able to eat or drink carbs, use a correction factor every 3–4 h.

Sick-Day Rules

Feeling under the weather? Follow these sick-day rules to help prevent dangerous blood glucose highs and diabetic ketoacidosis:

1. Check blood glucose every 2–3 h.
2. Continue taking basal and bolus insulin. If you don't feel like eating, try to drink your carbs so that you can prevent starvation ketones and continue to take mealtime insulin. If you can't eat, skip the meal bolus and take the correction bolus if glucose is >200 mg/dL.
3. Check blood or urine ketones frequently with a test strip. Have a plan in place with your provider or call your provider for what to do about any positive results.
4. Stay hydrated by drinking a cup of fluid every hour, keeping in mind that vomiting and diarrhea increase the risk of dehydration.

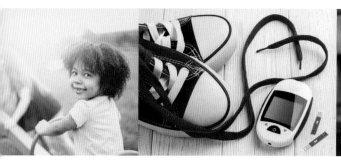
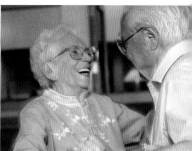

CHAPTER **8**

Physical Activity

Having type 1 diabetes doesn't mean that you can't win an Olympic gold medal or race in the Indianapolis 500. Or hike, bike, or skateboard. In this chapter, you'll learn how to be successful doing any sort of physical activity that you desire.

All people, with or without diabetes, benefit from physical activity and exercise. There are both short-term and long-term benefits: improved heart and lung fitness, increased muscle strength, weight control, improved balance and mobility, and better psychological health. Regular exercise reduces levels of bad LDL cholesterol and triglycerides, raises levels of good HDL cholesterol, and combats inflammation. Together, these improvements can lower the risk of heart attacks and strokes.

But as good as it can be for you or your child, in some ways exercise can make type 1 diabetes management harder, particularly when you start a new exercise program. Exercise can increase the risk of low blood glucose levels during and up to a day after the activity. It can also make blood glucose levels transiently too high.

During exercise, the muscles open up a special trap door—one that doesn't rely on insulin—to absorb glucose from the bloodstream. Low- and moderate-intensity exercise can therefore lower how much insulin you need to hit blood glucose targets. Aerobic exercise—jogging, walking, cycling, swimming—typically leads to a greater reduction than strength training.

There's No Way to Be "Perfect"

"Running with type 1 diabetes is always a complicated challenge. Since every run is different, your blood sugars will never act exactly the same each time. You'll go into the run with different amounts of food and insulin in your system, you'll run at different paces and start at different times, you'll run at different inclines or take different length breaks. The key is knowing you won't get it right every time and to keep checking your blood sugar to stay on top of any changes. A continuous glucose monitor makes running so much easier I can't imagine ever running without one.

For me, there is always a strong desire to eliminate as many variables as possible: waking up at the same time every day, eating the same thing for breakfast, working out at the same intensity. And while it will make parts of type 1 diabetes less complicated, you'll never be able to eliminate all the variables and, because of that, you'll never be able to eliminate all of the high and low blood sugars. Once I realized that there was no way to be 'perfect,' it let me stop feeling like that was something I had to strive towards. I could live my life the way I wanted to live it without letting type 1 diabetes dictate what I did or didn't do."

—Craig Stubing

Impetus and Understanding

"I can honestly say that physical exercise is the best control I have for maintaining my health. In tracking my blood sugars on a daily basis, when I am not taking care of my health because I am too busy to commit to the required exercise, my blood sugars are high and not in control. When I have followed a regular, moderate exercise program that features cardiovascular activity and other strengthening elements, my blood sugars are much more in control, I feel better, and I do not exhibit the symptoms of high blood sugars—fatigue, irritability, thirst. The effect of regular exercise gives me the impetus, understanding, and means to stop the daily decline and compromise of myself as a result of physical inactivity."

—Jay Stein, 68, is an attorney who regularly "manages" the
Los Angeles Dodgers from his offices and home.

"Donuts!"

"During one high school gym class, we stayed inside due to bad weather. We ended up running the hallways in the lower level to make up for the track running we were supposed to do outside. Turns out that the gym teacher didn't know the first thing about diabetes and the whole class, plus the teacher, found out what can happen to a T1D. While running around the hallways, keeping up with the class, I ran into severe hypoglycemia. I ended up on the floor, all white and pale skin. Knowing we had donuts waiting for us at the finish, I yelled out, 'I NEED some donuts!' With that, one classmate ran and got me a box from the table. After I brought my BG up, I told the nurse my story, and they created a new process for students with diabetes and specific gym routines planned for us."

—Robert Grass, 51, is a management consultant.
He can often be found hiking in the backcountry
of Angeles National Forest.

Hypoglycemia with Exercise

Preventing hypoglycemia (low blood glucose) is an essential part of a complete workout for people with type 1 diabetes. Hypoglycemia can occur during and immediately after physical activity, as well as over the next 24–48 h. Monitoring blood glucose and becoming familiar with your/your child's personal responses to exercise can help prevent immediate and delayed hypoglycemia.

To calculate how much to lower your insulin dose before an exercise session or how many extra carbs you need to eat to keep blood glucose from dipping too low, you'll need to consider the type of physical activity and the intensity at which you plan to exercise. Lengthy high-intensity aerobic activity is associated with the highest risk of going low.

High-intensity interval training—short bouts of super-intense exercise followed by longer recovery periods—is also associated with hypoglycemia. However, it can also cause an increase in blood glucose levels immediately after the intensive exercise phases. A little resistance training before aerobic exercise may actually prevent hypoglycemia, and cross training is just a good idea for general fitness. Check out Adam Brown's column at diaTribe.org for detailed guidelines and advice about exercise.

The best defense against exercise-related hypoglycemia is to prepare with some carbohydrates. How much varies by person, insulin regimen, and current blood glucose level, as well as the activity's type, timing, intensity, and duration. At least 10–15 g of fast-acting carbohydrates are recommended, but this is highly individual. Carefully follow blood glucose levels before, during, and after exercise and be prepared to treat.

People who are concerned about weight gain often complain of having to constantly eat after exercise to prevent low blood glucose levels. Discuss strategies with your/your child's diabetes health-care team on adjusting carb intake and insulin dosing for the meal prior to exercise as well as what to do with your/your child's insulin dosing during exercise.

> Different types of exercise will have different effects in terms of blood glucose levels. Exercise can both lower or raise blood glucose levels depending on the circumstances.

Hyperglycemia

People are often surprised when they start exercising and find that their blood glucose levels rise instead of fall. This happens when the body perceives exercise as an added stress, so adrenaline and other hormones come out to raise blood glucose levels. If you are just starting an exercise program and you join a spin class, at first your body struggles to keep up. Your blood glucose levels may rise. But over time your body gets fitter and the exercise is less stressful, so the stress hormones don't come out and blood glucose levels may fall with the same exercise. Intensity makes a difference: walking on flat ground for 60 min almost always lowers blood glucose levels, but hiking up a mountain for an hour may lower OR raise blood glucose levels. Your level of fitness can change over time. If you get sick or travel and stop exercising for a while, you may be a bit out of shape and find differences in how you respond to exercise.

Expect the unexpected, and be prepared. During competition, Olympian Gary Hall, Jr., would see his blood glucose rise because of the stress of the race from 150 to 350—in just 21 sec! That happened every time, except when it didn't, and very rarely his blood glucose level would be 35 at the end of a race.

So the answer is to be ready with rapid-acting carbohydrates even if you think your glucose will always be high after a certain exercise.

The biggest mistake people tend to make is to over-treat the high blood glucose after exercise. After a workout, the body needs to restore glucose into muscle (the muscle stores glucose as glycogen), and it is like a sponge sucking up water, whether the blood glucose level is high, low, or normal. This is a time when you need to give your body fuel (carbohydrates) and perhaps insulin, but use less insulin than usual (maybe half a dose, but discuss with your health-care team) to avoid immediate post-exercise rebound lows. But regardless of whether your blood glucose level is high after exercise, you are still at risk of lows 12–24 h later (often at night), so watch for this and adjust your overnight insulin dose as needed.

Certain types of high-intensity exercise, such as sprinting and powerlifting, can increase blood glucose levels in the short term. The body responds to anaerobic exercise by pumping up levels of stress hormones, which, among other functions, trigger the liver to pump out extra glucose to keep the muscles from becoming depleted. If you're in a competition, like a race, that stress can also trigger hyperglycemia. Trying too hard to prevent hypoglycemia—by over-consuming carbohydrates or withholding too much insulin—can also lead to a high. Illness and a blocked insulin pump may also be behind a seemingly exercise-related high. Going into exercise a little bit high is fine—exercise will likely take care of the situation.

Strategies such as doing a cooldown of light walking or cycling for 15–20 min after strenuous exercise can help lower blood glucose levels more gradually. Also, varying the timing of high-intensity exercise during the workout can also help prevent lows and highs.

Stay well hydrated during exercise, as dehydration can exacerbate highs. If you become dehydrated, you become resistant to the action of insulin and blood glucose levels can increase. It can also increase the risk of leg cramps. Drink enough fluids when competing or exercising for longer periods of time, such as running a marathon. Some sports drinks contain sugar and electrolytes, often good to use before or during exercise. Others contain some protein as well, which are promoted as recovery drinks. Most people who exercise for fitness do not need to be "serious" about the various types of fluid for hydration. More serious athletes will learn for themselves what is most effective.

HOW MUCH EXERCISE DO WE NEED?

Infants and toddlers: Encouraging infants to explore movement and their surroundings supports physical and mental development, as does active play. For toddlers, ≥30 min more of physical activity a day with ≤60 min of sitting at a time will promote motor skills and muscular development.

Preschoolers should bump up their physical activity to ≥60 min per day. Give your child 5–15 g of carbohydrates for every 30 min of activity, depending on initial blood glucose levels and the intensity of the exercise. Supervising adults will want to check pre-exercise blood glucose levels in active young children because they may not be able to verbalize the symptoms of a low. Starting exercise with blood glucose in the 150–200-mg/dL range may help lower the risk of hypoglycemia in toddlers.

Children and adolescents: Children and adolescents need ≥60 min of physical activity each day. Both aerobic activities and anaerobic activities should be included, as well as strength training, such as yoga, light weights, and other activities.

Exercise is important for overall fitness, but so is limiting the amount of time sitting. Kids these days tend to spend a lot of time in front of various screens—television, computers, video games, tablets, smartphones, and so on. Too much screen time is associated with higher blood glucose levels, while physical activity is linked to lower A1Cs and healthier hearts. Experts recommend limiting sedentary time to <2 h per day.

The tricky part about exercise in children of all ages is that it is often unplanned and spontaneous. Today, will your child come home from school and do homework for an hour or want to bike with friends for an hour? Sometimes you don't know if they are going to run around for just 15 min or keep running around for an hour and need extra carbs to prevent a low. Be prepared to give 5–15 g of carbs, depending on the child's age and size, for every 30 min of sustained activity and monitor glucose levels frequently.

> Any type of exercise is better than no exercise, but be sure to start slow and build up to avoid injury.

Adults: Experts recommend that people aged 18–64 years work out aerobically at a moderate or vigorous pace for ≥150 min per week, adding in a couple of strength-training sessions, such as lifting weights or kettlebells, or doing yoga, for extra fitness. With exercise, some is good and more is better. The American College of Sports Medicine recommends that adults burn ~1,000 calories per week, the amount it takes to walk at a moderate pace for ~5 h—though expending only 500 calories per week still has its benefits.

If exercise is a new thing for you, start slowly and work up. Some exercise beats no exercise every time. Don't get fixated on joining fancy gyms or signing up for aerial yoga classes (though they are pretty cool). Start out with something simple. Grab a coworker and walk for 15–20 min during your lunch hour. Too busy at work? Grab a friend, spouse, neighbor, or even a pet and walk after dinner.

Break up periods of sitting with moving. Exercising every night for an hour does not negate the harms caused by sitting all day long. So every day should consist of periods of sitting interspersed with moving. Set an alarm to go off every hour, vow to always walk around when talking on the phone, or get a mini portable treadmill to put under your desk. Just move, and then move some more!

The number one reason adults give for not exercising? Not enough time. But physical activity doesn't need to involve a time-consuming trip to the gym. Gardening, playing sports, bike commuting, taking the stairs, and other blood pumping activities still count toward your goal. For adults with type 1 diabetes, the benefits of exercise—such as reducing the risk of heart attacks, strokes, early death, certain types of cancer, and osteoporosis—far exceed the risks.

A big myth about exercise is that it leads to weight loss. Until you exercise intensively for ≥ 2 h per day, exercise does not cause weight loss. A combination of eating less and exercising more causes weight loss. People who exercise are often those more focused on health, so exercise can be a sign that someone is on a healthy path, but by itself exercise won't reduce weight. In fact it often makes people more hungry, and then the additional calories will negate any possibility of losing weight.

Older adults: For older adults, the exercise recommendations are generally the same as for other adults—150 min aerobic activity per week, plus two strengthening sessions. There are a few extra considerations:

- Chronic conditions such as arthritis can get in the way of reaching the target amount of physical activity, but it's still beneficial to get as close to those goals as abilities and conditions allow.
- Falls are a serious risk of older adults; complications from falls can limit mobility and make it even more difficult to keep up with the activities required for daily living. Exercises that maintain and improve balance—such as yoga, Pilates, and balance training—can reduce the risk of falls.
- If you have health issues that make it more challenging to exercise, talk with a health-care provider or exercise physiologist with type 1 diabetes experience.

See **Table 8.1** for a summary of activities.

Elite Athletes

It is clear that having type 1 diabetes doesn't have to stop people from performing at elite levels. However, it does add complexity to training and competing. Ideally a person training for an event should learn what the general drill consists of—how people without diabetes train, because this is likely to be a good guide as to what is metabolically required, and then it can be modified for the person with type 1 diabetes.

There are many resources for athletes with type 1 diabetes and often the best guides are people with type 1 diabetes who have been competing in the same events. Trading tips and strategies can be very helpful, as can finding others train-

TABLE 8.1   Get the Right Amount of Activity for Your Age

Age (years)	Minimum Activity	Details
0–4	30–60 min/d	Indoor and outdoor activities that encourage motor skill development.
5–18	60 min/d	• Vigorous-intensity aerobics at ≥3 days a week • Muscle and bone-strengthening activities ≥3 days a week
18–64	150 moderate to vigorous aerobic activity minutes/ week + 2 days resistance training/ week	• Perform activity in sessions lasting ≥10 min • Don't go more than 2 consecutive days without activity
≥65	150 moderate aerobic activity minutes/week + 2 days resistance training/ week	• If chronic conditions limit activity, continue to exercise as much as is feasible • Select activities that maintain or improve balance to reduce risk of falling

---

Activity Basics

Discuss your plans with your health-care provider if you plan to substantially change exercise habits.

Be prepared and expect variability.

Have a plan for treating highs and lows.

Wear appropriate gear/footwear.

Have diabetes ID.

Be sure to have easy access to blood glucose monitoring, simple carbohydrates, and fluids.

Be slow and steady as you increase to your goals.

Hydrate.

Monitor.

Use carbs and insulin to maintain steady numbers, understanding the balance.

Set goals.

Learn from experience; be aware of the training effect and how it can influence your blood glucose values.

ing for the same event who can become training buddies. Having a health-care team who are experienced in working with athletes who have type 1 diabetes can also be very helpful—including an expert nutritionist, exercise physiologist, and potentially a sports psychologist.

Preexisting Conditions

The value of exercise for people with type 1 diabetes is hard to overstate; however, diabetes-related complications of the eyes, nerves, kidneys, and heart can increase the risks associated with physical activity. Taking certain precautions is warranted.

Heart Disease or Stroke

Type 1 diabetes raises the risk of blood vessel damage, which can trigger heart attacks or strokes. The longer your duration of diabetes, the higher this risk. If you have had type 1 for >10–15 years and are aged ≥30 years, undergo a screening by a physician or qualified exercise professional (e.g., ACSM-certified exercise physiologist) before starting a new exercise program. You may also be asked whether you've experience any warning signs of heart disease, such as:

- Difficulty completing normal activities
- Shortness of breath
- Lack of energy
- Shoulder pain
- Activity-related dizziness
- Fatigue
- Neck or jaw discomfort
- Upper back pain

If you have any of these symptoms, which could be symptoms of heart disease, you may need to undergo cardiac testing to be sure your heart can handle the increase in exercise.

Retinopathy

There is concern that increases in blood pressure and jarring activities may damage blood vessels in the eye in people with advanced retinopathy, a vision-threatening complication of diabetes. If you have advanced eye disease, avoid activities that raise systolic blood pressure to >170 mmHg, such as weightlifting and extra vigorous aerobic activity. Most people with diabetic eye disease can (and should) exercise. Discuss appropriate limits with your eye care professional, especially if you are being treated with laser or injections into your eyes or have had recent eye surgery.

Neuropathy

Diabetes-related nerve damage can cause weakness, pain, and numbness in the feet and other body parts. Staying on top of foot care, preventing falls, and screening for nerve-related heart conditions are important precautions for people with neuropathy. But exercise remains, overall, a healthy choice, and it can actually help prevent neuropathy and foot ulcers in those with neuropathy, according to some data. The key points here are to "mind your feet":

- Always wear clean socks.
- Wear shoes that fit well. You may need special shoes prescribed by your provider and fitted by a specialist.
- Wash your feet and check for any damage from shoes and exercise.

If you have nerve damage to your feet (numbness, tingling, shooting pains) you may need to see a foot doctor (podiatrist) for regular check-ups. Diabetic foot ulcers don't happen suddenly—they happen because small blisters or sores are overlooked. So check your feet every day and report any changes to your health-care provider. You are the keeper of your feet and they will thank you for your attention! For people with more advanced disease, supervised exercise may help prevent falls and injury. In some cases, special shoes can help protect the feet and improve mobility.

Nephropathy

It is generally OK to exercise if you have kidney disease, but be extra careful not to get dehydrated. It is likely that you will be on blood pressure medications if you have kidney disease, and this may impact your blood pressure while exercising. Discuss your exercise plans with your health-care provider, and be sure to report if you feel dizzy or light-headed.

SPECIAL ACTIVITIES

Scuba Diving

People with type 1 diabetes used to be counseled against scuba diving because of a fear that they would become hypoglycemic underwater and not be able to ascend quickly enough to treat a low. Now, however, with a physician's clearance, scuba diving is permitted as long as certain safety precautions are followed. Generally these include diving when the blood glucose level is higher rather than lower, diving with a partner who is aware of the diabetes, and carrying glucose gels for treatment if hypoglycemia occurs. Diving is a form of physical activity, so blood glucose levels can fall. Patients have successfully dived all around the world. Go to ddrc.org/DivingDiabetes for more information.

Skydiving

Mothers and doctors may blanch at the thought, but people with type 1 diabetes can skydive. If you are not an experienced skydiver, the adrenaline of the jump and fall will raise your blood glucose levels. You must make sure that all of your diabetes devices are well secured so they don't fall to earth when you jump out of the plane.

Barbados to Japan

"I was diagnosed with T1D when I was 18 years old. Now I am 19, a professional stand-up paddle racer/surfer and windsurfer, and competing the majority of the year. In the past 6 months I've competed and traveled to 10 countries, from Barbados to Japan to France, and just about everywhere in between. Life isn't necessarily easy with T1D, but it's different. I am still doing everything I was doing before, but now it takes more planning. I have learned to pay much more attention to my body and in return, I feel that I have become healthier. My optimum range to start a surf session or competition is 160–175. I always bring fast-acting glucose with me when I go out on the water. Then I'm ready for a fun session!

Remember that T1D is a process and it takes time to figure everything out, but you will. You will find a rhythm. If it isn't going perfect, take a big breath, don't stress, and start to fix your blood sugar. You got this!"

—Fiona Wylde was the 2016 Stand-Up Paddle Racing world champion.

Surfing

In Southern California, surfing is a common activity. Many adolescents and young adults spend many summertime hours in the ocean. Using a patch pump or even a sensor is difficult because they come off with too much exposure to salt water. Some pumps with tubing have to be taken off and left on shore and are hard to use if surfing all day long. A hybrid solution can be worked out. Some people give an injection of rapid- or short-acting insulin before eating and then go surf, without a pump, and then put the pump back on when out of the water. Others use an injection regimen over the summer and go back on the pump in the fall. Work this out with your health-care team. Of note, insulin can be overheated and become less active if left in the sun or on the beach for too long, and it can also go bad if left uncooled in a hot car. Store insulin in a cooling container (but not on ice).

Hiking, Backpacking, Rock Climbing, Mountaineering

People with type 1 diabetes have hiked, trekked, and climbed all over the world. Bring double or triple the amount of insulin and supplies you think you might need and make sure some of it is always carried on your body as well as on the body of a friend. Consider this case: a woman went snowboarding in the wilderness and had her boyfriend carry her insulin in his parka while she carried her meter. He lost his way and went down a ravine, and search and rescue took 2 days to find him. She had to wait for 2 days in a remote wilderness outpost and nearly went into serious DKA before insulin could be obtained.

Consider the effects of heat, cold, and altitude on insulin, meters, and glucose test strips, and the changes in insulin requirements physical activity may cause.

Prepare for potential ailments—bring antibiotics to take for skin infections and diarrhea (as recommended by your health-care team), get all needed vaccines (see a travel specialist if going to the developing world), and be sure to bring something to treat nausea and vomiting as well as oral rehydration tablets. When people get dehydrated, especially if it is from a sickness such as a diarrheal illness, being able to drink fluids with water and electrolytes can make a huge difference.

Race Car Driving

Race car driving is an inherently dangerous activity, but with proper preparation, type 1 diabetes does not need to be a hindrance. Avoiding lows (which could cause harm to other drivers), wearing a continuous glucose monitor, and having glucose solution available at all times are central to safe driving. For any professional sport, you will want to create an expert team to help guide every aspect of training and competing.

Olympic Competition

Gary Hall, Jr., is an Olympic swimmer who won four medals before he had type 1 diabetes and six medals in two Olympics after he was diagnosed. He is an outstanding example of what is possible. However, he, as do all elite athletes, faces certain additional challenges due to having type 1 diabetes. Two issues encountered by highly skilled athletes are the negative effects of insulin resistance and ketosis caused by illness or stress preventing optimal race preparation, as well as the negative effects of nighttime hypoglycemia just before an event. As with race car drivers, working closely with a team consisting of individuals from a variety of disciplines, as well as connecting with athletes who have performed in similar events, can be very helpful. In the specific instance of Gary Hall, Jr., there were times when his diabetes impacted his swimming, but he never once blamed his diabetes for a poor performance. And overall, his natural talent and competitive mindset were able to rise above any challenges caused by his diabetes. From the start, he figured out how to treat his diabetes in a way that worked for him—an approach that still works well for him now that he is in his 40s.

A Whole New Strength

"Over my 13 years of diabetes—11 of those exercising regularly and 9 doing endurance sports—I've found that exercise with diabetes is a constant challenge that rewards you tenfold.

I started running because I needed to fulfill a college gym requirement. Over time I realized that it was a good way to clear my head, feel strong, and lower my blood sugar levels. Eventually, I discovered the joy of overcoming obstacles through endurance racing. To date I have racked up more than two dozen marathons, century rides, triathlons, and 5K swims.

Why spend all those hours of my life willingly subjecting myself to pain and boredom instead of lying on the couch watching TV?

Physically, I feel healthier. My A1C is at its best when I'm training, which means vigorous exercise 5 days a week. I feel safer for the future, knowing that I am keeping my circulatory system strong against complications. Unexpectedly, the more I exercise the more energy I have—I feel sluggish and drink twice as much coffee when I don't work out for a few days.

Mentally, my head feels clearer after a good workout. I can manage negative emotions and amplify positive ones. Finding workout buddies and teammates means that I have made new friends and forged deep connections, even raising money for diabetes organizations (including Tour de Cure).

You have to experiment and be patient. Record blood glucose levels and insulin doses for a couple of days and see what trends you spot. Try different fuel options on a long run. Know that as your body becomes more sensitive to insulin, things may change in just a few weeks. Also, be safe. It's okay to ramp up slowly as you figure out how your body responds. Look for creative gear options to always bring your meter, insulin, and glucose with you, whether it's a backpack or pocket or belt. Make exercise as fun as possible if you don't naturally enjoy it. It's essential to have at least a little fun if you're going to make it a habit—even if the only part you enjoy is listening to music or watching a TV show while you move. Experiment with different ways to make it fun, and leave behind the forms of exercise that feel like a total drag.

By working out, especially through endurance athletics, I find a whole new strength. When my body feels broken or defective from diabetes, exercise is a way to show the world that my body can do truly amazing things. It means that my spirit is strong enough to overcome challenges and adapt to the never-ending challenges of diabetes. For every time I feel weak, depressed, or discouraged, I can think of a time when I felt capable and powerful. Making exercise a habit is my way of saying I am stronger than diabetes."

—Caroline Sheehan, 30, is a case manager and sings soprano in her church's gospel choir.

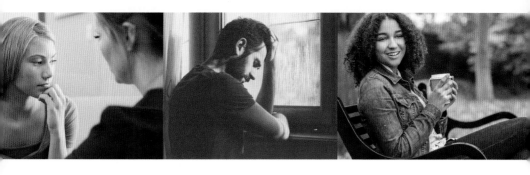

CHAPTER 9

Mental Health

Tracking blood glucose levels, dosing insulins, planning your meals, and taking care of your physical needs are vital. So is maintaining your mental and emotional health. Feeling good is more than half the battle—feeling good about yourself allows you to take care of yourself.

People with type 1 diabetes are at a heightened risk of psychosocial issues, including diabetes distress, depression, anxiety, and disordered eating, but these are all treatable disorders. It is important to pay attention to your feelings about having diabetes or taking care of someone who has diabetes, and the barriers to good treatment. Talk to your physician, your diabetes educator—anyone you connect with on your diabetes team. They can help set you up with mental health care as needed, whether it is with a counselor, a therapist, a psychiatrist, or a social worker. Having support in living with diabetes is essential.

One issue with diabetes is that it is a very "numeric" disease—it is easy to measure blood glucose levels and an A1C and then tie an emotion to the number. Many patients come into a doctor's office and anxiously await their A1C number to see if they are doing well or poorly. But diabetes is far more than a number, it is a condition that influences individuals' and families' lives. This influence can be both negative and positive. Find the success in your diabetes management. If you were checking your blood glucose levels only twice a day last month but checked four times a day this month and gave insulin more consistently, that is a win, regardless of your A1C.

Every day there are triumphs in managing your diabetes. Look at variability—how much your blood glucose levels go up and down in a day. It is a success when the variability is reduced, even if your A1C is the same. You are not "bad" or inadequate if your blood glucose levels are sometimes out of range. High blood glucose levels are correctable; the bigger issue is when people give up trying. And that is where mental health issues come into play.

Tough on Perfectionists

"I discovered I had type 1 diabetes at age 35. My Type A personality did not take well to the news. I was a competitive, high-achieving, impatient, deadline-driven, goal-oriented, conscientious, self-critical perfectionist.

I found out that having diabetes is pretty tough on perfectionists.

At first, I tried to do everything my doctor and nutritionist told me to do. I gave multiple daily injections and pricked my fingers several times a day. I carried around a fat paperback book that listed the carb count of thousands of foods (it was the pre-iPhone era) and looked up everything I was about to eat, just ate, or thought about eating. I bought a larger purse to accommodate the carb counting book as well as all the testing and insulin supplies. I kept detailed logs; I changed the timing and intensity of my exercise routines; I woke up in the middle of the night to correct lows or highs.

But no matter how 'good' I was, there were always lows and highs I couldn't explain. After just a few months, I became overwhelmed, frustrated, and discouraged. I decided I didn't want to deal with my diabetes any longer.

Not a good move.

Luckily, after not too long, my doctor gave me the name of a therapist. Skeptical at first, I eventually attended a workshop. That day turned out to be one of the most significant experiences in my life. The therapist homed in on one issue that made a lot of sense to me: the Type A thing. Knowing I had been a straight A student, he asked whether I felt I was trying to achieve an A in diabetes.

This changed my entire perspective. I realized I had been ignoring my diabetes so I wouldn't constantly be reminded that I was failing at something. But the therapist helped me see that I was actually doing a really good job managing my diabetes. I still took my insulin every day, looked up carb content, and tested my BGs every now and then. He reassured me that diabetes is tricky and can't always be managed perfectly, but that I was definitely doing a good job trying.

At the end of the workshop, the therapist handed me a piece of paper with an A written on it. I've now had diabetes for 12 years—and I'm still getting an A!"

—Debra Grossman, 47, is an attorney
and has two children.

> Diabetes distress is different from depression, and is an understandable response to the demands of living with type 1 diabetes.

DIABETES DISTRESS

We once thought that people with type 1 diabetes had more depression than other people, and while research is divided about that, it is clear that the much more common problem is diabetes distress. Depression is an illness that anyone can develop, and it is treated with medication and therapy. Diabetes distress isn't a medical problem; it is the understandable stress that comes from living day in and day out with the challenge of managing diabetes. Diabetes distress can affect both you and your family, and it can change over time.

Do you feel burned out by the constant effort it takes to manage diabetes? Do you feel upset, guilty, or anxious if your diabetes management or that of your child is off track? Please discuss this with your health-care team. In particular, a therapist or a diabetes educator (or both) can help you find solutions. You may be given a questionnaire to pinpoint where you are having the most trouble. Two surveys that are often used are the Problem Areas in Diabetes Questionnaire (PAID) and the Diabetes Distress Scale (DDS).

People with diabetes distress need support and perhaps specific skills for coping with diabetes. All people can learn to cope with diabetes though there are phases when it is easier and harder to deal with.

I Don't Want to Wonder

"Find the reason to take care of your diabetes, a reason that extends beyond the basic desire to avoid complications or to maintain a good A1C. For me, that is to perform my best academically and athletically. With the technologies available today, there is no reason that I need to allow diabetes to affect my performance. I don't want to wonder years from now what I could have been capable of if I had been more diligent about my diabetes control. I don't see diabetes as an excuse, rather a challenge that I'm capable of handling. For someone else, this motivation might be to be a good role model for a loved one or to have success in your career. I find that having this larger motivation has saved me from the ever-present danger of 'diabetes burn-out.' There are still many times when I know I could do a better job, but keeping my larger goals in mind helps to bring me back on track."

— Delaney Miller, 20, is an NCAA Division I track athlete at Princeton. She has had diabetes since the age of 4.

> Depression is a treatable medical issue—be sure to speak with someone from your health care team if you find your mood interferes with your ability to function.

DEPRESSION

We can all get down in the dumps sometimes, but when feelings of sadness are persistent and get in the way of living life, that's depression, a serious mood disorder. Apart from the general mental and physical toll depression can take, people with type 1 diabetes have additional concerns that may make them more at risk of depression.

Overall, the symptoms of depression involve changes in weight (eating too much or too little), feeling blue, sleeping too much or too little, and not finding enjoyment in life or activities. These are fairly nonspecific. However, if your mood is interfering with your ability to take care of yourself or function day to day, you need to ask for help.

Depression can look different in a teenager. Teenagers who are depressed can have declining school performance, withdrawal from friends and activities, anger, agitation, and/or irritability.

Depression can be related to age and life events such as loss of a job or a loved one. A family history of depression increases the risk, as does having low self-esteem and social support. People with type 1 diabetes may be most vulnerable for depression at these times:

- Adolescence
- End of diabetes "honeymoon" period
- During treatment intensification
- At a hospitalization
- The development or progression of complications
- Pregnancy
- Life changes (marriage, divorce, loss of job)
- Problems with glucose control or insulin regimen

Many clinics now screen patients for depression at their regular visits with the PHQ 2 Questionnaire **(Table 9.1)**. It is just two questions. If the answer to either is "nearly every day" or "more than half the days," then a longer test is given. People who score in the range of depression should receive treatment. Depression can be effectively treated by medication, psychotherapy, or both.

Researchers have noted a correlation between type 1 diabetes, depression, and worsening health. The connection seems not to be a direct biological link between depression and blood glucose levels, but rather that depression may make it more difficult to successfully engage in the self-care behavior that type 1 demands. The evidence for the role of self-management is spotty in adults, but one study in adolescents with type 1 diabetes found that a good portion of the relationship between A1C levels and depression could be explained by the frequency of blood glucose monitoring. In other words, teenagers who experience depressive symptoms check blood glucose less frequently than those without depression, which leads to higher average blood glucose levels. Overall, it is clear that poor outcomes in people with type 1 diabetes are interrelated with depression. That is why a whole-person approach to type 1 care is essential; the body and mind are one.

TABLE 9.1   Patient Health Questionnaire-2: Screening Instrument for Depression

Over the past two weeks, how often have you been bothered by any of the following problems?	Not at all	Several days	More than half the days	Nearly every day
Little interest or pleasure in doing things	0	1	2	3
Feeling down, depressed, or hopeless	0	1	2	3

Eating disorders are more common in females with type 1 diabetes and need to be diagnosed and treated if they exist.

EATING DISORDERS

The pressures to be thin can feel overbearing in our society, and women and girls with type 1 diabetes are at an elevated risk of eating disorders compared to those without the disease. There is basically no data on eating disorders in men and boys with type 1 diabetes. However, disordered eating does occur among men and boys in the general population, so don't ignore warning signs.

Eating disorders are common among women and girls in the general population; however, those with type 1 are around twice as likely to suffer from disordered eating patterns. These can include inappropriate dieting for weight loss, binge eating, or purging through vomiting, laxative or diuretic use, excessive exercise, or through insulin restriction. This final behavior is specific to type 1 diabetes and can be extremely dangerous.

Women with type 1 diabetes and eating disorders have, on average, A1Cs that are 2% higher than those without eating disorders. People with type 1 diabetes who have diagnosable eating disorders tend to have higher rates of diabetes distress and fear of hypoglycemia. Hospitalization rates, emergency room visits, neuropathy, retinopathy, and the risk of premature death are also elevated in women with eating disorders.

Why does type 1 diabetes predispose women to eating disorders? No one knows for sure. Anyone who has high blood glucose levels over a period of days to weeks knows that higher blood glucose levels lead to weight loss and controlled blood glucose levels can cause weight gain. Type 1 diabetes also encourages dietary micromanagement. In the general population, paying very close attention to food portions is linked to an increased risk of eating disorders.

Warning Signs of Eating Disorders

- Unexplained increase in A1C levels
- Repeated episodes of DKA
- Extreme concerns of body size/shape
- Excessive exercise and related hypoglycemia
- Very low-calorie meals
- Absence of menstruation

Diabulimia

Diabulimia is often used to describe an eating disorder that centers on intentionally restricting insulin to stimulate weight loss. The result is high levels of glucose in the blood that spill over into the urine, leading to the excretion of the calories from glucose. The repercussions can be severe, including dehydration, loss of lean body tissue, and, in extreme cases, DKA. Diabulimia is shockingly common; as many as a third of women with type 1 diabetes report insulin restriction, with higher levels among those between the ages of 15 and 30.

Once insulin restriction or other disordered eating behaviors become engrained, a cycle of shame, guilt, and other negative feelings can make it difficult to get help and the condition difficult to treat. A team-based approach is the gold standard, with inclusion of a mental health professional along with the other team members (endocrinologist, nurse educator, nutritionist, etc.). In severe cases, hospitalization may be necessary until mental and medical stability are achieved. Monthly or more frequent appointments with members of the care team may be needed.

I Knew How to Play the Game

"As a type 1 diabetic from the age of 7, I just knew I was an expert on this disease. I rolled my eyes at countless nurses, endocrinologists, and educators who lectured me endlessly on ways to manage my diabetes. I could mix water with my blood and get a perfect reading on my meter every time. I wore a pump. I even got out of traffic tickets from officers using 'insulin pump emergencies' as an excuse. I was invincible. No doctor or nurse or anyone could tell me any differently, especially if they didn't have to live with it. How dare they?

My A1C, however, was through the roof. I had multiple retinopathy surgeries to stop the bleeding in my eyes, I only had four toes left, and yet, diabulimia was still strong. I lay in ICU on an insulin drip thinking, 'I have got to get out of here and off this drip; I'm getting fatter by the minute.' I was so focused on carbohydrates and food and insulin, all day, every day—but not for the right reasons. I knew how to play the food-medicine game. I could eat anything I wanted and then some, and lose weight. I would live at my threshold, taking the tiniest basal amounts of insulin just to skirt by, exhausted and thirsty. I could hardly function day to day.

I had all these complications and forgot what it meant to feel good. I was an angry and sad person. The ignorance of the public, my friends, and some of my family was frustrating and hurtful. I felt I was being blamed. Oh, the stigma of having diabetes, "the fat people's disease." The comments still ring in my head to this day: 'You don't look like a diabetic,' I would hear. 'If you just ate the right things; exercise it away,' they would say.

When I was pregnant, I was singularly focused on having a healthy pregnancy, bringing my A1C down to 5.6. But after my daughter was born, I didn't want to gain weight, so I started cutting insulin again.

I was sacrificing my entire life to diabulimia, until my daughter was diagnosed at the age of 2 with type 1 diabetes. I was sick over it. And the comments: 'If you just fed her right...' or 'Maybe she will outgrow it...' Then it hit me. I cannot let her grow up feeling the same way I did: alone, frustrated, misunderstood, and judged.

More than anything, I wanted her to enjoy her life, which had just begun, and I wanted to be alive and well enough to get her to adulthood. I wanted to be a great *mother but I was too tired to play, too sick to give her all the attention she deserved. She made toes for me out of Play-Doh so I could chase her at the playground. She looked up to me for guidance. Did she think this was her future?*

We were a team. We would fight it together. I would not let her down. Screw this disease and everything it had already taken from me. I refused to let it now take her mother from her."

—Kathlin Gordon, 40, is a registered dietitian nutritionist.

DIABETES DISTRESS THROUGH THE LIFE SPAN

Infants, Young Children, and Parents

For parents there is often an overwhelming sense of responsibility and guilt—"How did I cause this?"—and failure—"Why can't my son have perfect blood sugar levels when I try so hard?" Parents often have a lot of worry and anxiety about hypoglycemia, especially overnight. They are often up a lot at night checking blood glucose levels and therefore are sleep deprived. It is common for these parents to have anxiety, higher distress levels, and even depression after the diabetes diagnosis and even down the road. If you are having these feelings, please reach out to your diabetes team for help and support. Gaining their support and educating other adults connected with your child on the important basics of your child's diabetes will help you, your child, and others who want to ensure the best life experiences for your child.

You may have concerns about parenting and discipline. It's natural to feel sorry for your child who is living with diabetes, and it's common to be more lenient with typical toddler behavior because of this. Parents often describe behavior changes with low and high blood glucose levels, which complicates the decision to discipline bad behavior. Try to not negotiate diabetes-related tasks. If it is time to check a blood glucose or get an injection, do not allow the child to delay it with whining, debate, or tantrums. Consistency is important and will prevent the behaviors from escalating. It is important to reward and reinforce children when they work to subscribe to their diabetes management tasks. Reinforcing positive behaviors and decisions can go a long way to helping to ingrain in your child more optimal decisions throughout their lives.

Children

I'm Not Diabetes!

"After three years of going to camp and meeting others who don't mind walking around with a pump connected to their waist and their site in their arm or leg, it has shown me that I don't have to worry about what others possibly think. Everyone with diabetes probably has something that they hate about it. We all have the hard times, but most of the time, we can find silver linings from the most painful parts. Probably for me one of my biggest pet peeves is when someone

comes up to me and says, 'I feel so bad for you, since you have a DISEASE and have to give yourself shots all the time.' I HATE getting defined that I have a disease! I'm not diabetes, I'm ME!"

—Ayla Oceanna Kanow, 13, a competitive soccer player,
has had diabetes since age 9.

As kids grow older, the family learns to walk a fine line between the parent taking all of the responsibility for care and the growing child becoming independent. You worry about your child's health on a daily basis. Most parents don't have these same concerns. No wonder it causes distress! This transition period is challenging for many families. Getting enough support during these times from your diabetes health-care team, family, and even vital peers is important.

In some families, a parent and a child (or children) will have type 1 diabetes and diabetes management is truly a "family affair." However, each individual processes diabetes stresses differently and will need their own help in dealing with whatever issues they come across.

As children move through the various developmental stages of youth, certain family issues may arise **(Table 9.2)**. Your child's primary care provider is trained to look for and identify mental health issues that may arise and to know when to refer the patient for additional help. Some signs that a child is struggling and may need to see a mental health professional include:

• Sudden difficulty adhering to a diabetes care plan
• Frequent low and high blood glucose levels or DKA
• Academic issues
• Lying

Once your child reaches 12 years of age, your health-care provider should begin routine screening for depression **(Table 9.1)**.

TABLE 9.2   Childhood Life Stages, Issues, and Type 1 Diabetes

Developmental stages (ages)	Normal developmental tasks	T1D management priorities	Family issues in T1D management
Infancy (0–12 months)	Developing a trusting relationship or bonding with primary caregiver(s)	Preventing and treating hypoglycemia Avoiding extreme fluctuations in blood glucose levels.	Coping with stress Sharing the burden of care to avoid parent burnout
Toddler (13–26 months)	Developing a sense of mastery and autonomy	Preventing hypoglycemia Avoiding extreme fluctuations in blood glucose levels due to irregular food intake	Establishing a schedule Managing the picky eater Setting limits and coping with toddler's lack of cooperation with regimen Sharing the burden of care

TABLE 9.2   Childhood Life Stages, Issues, and Type 1 Diabetes (*Cont.*)

Developmental stages (ages)	Normal developmental tasks	T1D management priorities	Family issues in T1D management
Preschooler and early elementary school (3–7 years)	Developing initiative in activities and confidence in self	Preventing hypoglycemia Coping with unpredictable appetite and activity Positively reinforcing cooperation with regimen Trusting other caregivers with diabetes management	Reassuring child that diabetes is no one's fault Educating other caregivers about diabetes management
Older elementary school age (8–11 years)	Developing skills in athletic, cognitive, artistic, and social areas Consolidating self-esteem with respect to the peer group	Making diabetes regimen flexible to allow for participation in school or peer activities Child learning short- and long-term benefits of optimal management	Maintaining parental involvement in insulin and blood glucose monitoring tasks while allowing for independent self-care for special occasions Continuing to educate school and other caregivers
Early adolescence (12–15 years)	Managing body changes Developing a strong sense of self-identity	Increasing insulin requirements during puberty Diabetes management and blood glucose management becoming more difficult Weight and body image concerns	Renegotiating parent and teen's roles in diabetes management to be acceptable to both Learning coping skills to enhance ability to self-manage Preventing and intervening in diabetes-related family conflict Monitoring for signs of depression, eating disorders, risky behaviors
Later adolescence (16–19 years)	Establishing a sense of identity after high school (decisions about location, social issues, work, education)	Beginning an ongoing discussion of transition to a new diabetes team (discussion may begin in earlier adolescent years) Integrating diabetes into new lifestyle	Supporting the transition to independence Learning coping skills to enhance ability to self-manage Preventing and intervening with diabetes-related family conflict Monitoring for signs of depression, eating disorders, risky behaviors

Finding support and comfort from others living with type 1 diabetes can be a very positive experience.

Transitioning Youth

The transition from adolescence into adulthood (ages 18–30 years), sometimes referred to as "emerging adulthood," is a vulnerable period in the lives of people with type 1 diabetes. This stage is notoriously associated with blood glucose levels that are less balanced, and the reason isn't physical—it's psychosocial. During this part of life, a person typically moves out on their own for the first time. In addition to all the normal increases in responsibilities, the young adult with type 1 diabetes is suddenly fully in charge of managing a chronic disease. This flood of burden can trigger depressive symptoms, as well as eating disorders, anxiety, and fear of hypoglycemia. Preparing for this transition and getting additional help is key to making the jump to full adulthood as smooth as possible.

Happy Hour

"Living with type 1 diabetes became much easier—and I dare say even fun—once I started connecting in person with other people who had type 1 diabetes. Being able to sit at a happy hour with a dozen other people going through the same things every day that you're going through helps to disconnect from the bad days. You'll no longer feel like you did something wrong; you'll realize that bad days happen to everyone, so it can't just be because of you. Having people you can commiserate with when you're having a rough day will show you that even though you're the one managing your diabetes, you're not alone in the struggle."

—Craig Stubing

Adults

Diabetes self-management education is designed to help you deal with the trials and tribulations of a chronic disease. Make sure your needs are being met by talking to your educator or provider about any symptoms you're experiencing that may be related to depression or anxiety.

What you need will change over the decades. Usually (but not always) the late 20s and 30s are about settling down, starting a family, raising small children. This is a busy and disruptive time, especially for women who must have exceedingly tight blood glucose management during pregnancy and then act as caregivers. As people enter their 40s and 50s, life may be more settled, and there may be more time for diabetes self-care, although there is often time spent serving as a caregiver for an aging parent. As people become older still, they often develop other illnesses, such as heart disease, which make diabetes management more complicated and depression more common.

Time Travel

"An advantage to being diagnosed with sugar diabetes at the age of 3 is that you accept having a shot once a day as normal. I used to think that my friends that didn't have daily shots were unusual. In the early years the only way I could test for sugar levels at home was with Clinitest tablets. A jade green, opaque glass teacup, an eye dropper, and test tube were my set. Pee in the cup, put a tablet in the test tube, add a number of drops of urine and wait to see what color it turned after fizzing for a minute. Blue was good. Orange was bad. Later I retired the old cup and started peeing on test strips. They had more colors so you could make a better guess.

The first serious low I remember was when I was around 6 or 7. I had been to a movie by myself. The theater was next to my grandfather's barber shop. I was standing in a long line at the snack counter after the movie. I knew I was going low and needed a snack. I remember being jostled by other noisy impatient kids and just feeling out of it. When I finally got to the counter the attendant said, 'What do you want?' I replied, 'I don't know.' He told me to get out. My grandfather found me wandering around in front of the theater and took care of me. I realize now that there was always someone watching out for me even if I wasn't aware of it. As a parent I now realize just what a huge burden it was for my parents to make sure I had a 'normal' life.

Never in my life have I felt like I suffered from a disability. This is just the way life is. This is who I am, scars and all. My parents, at least when I was little, were the ones who suffered. I think when time travel is perfected, I'll go back and tell them everything is going to be all right."

—Drew Wickman

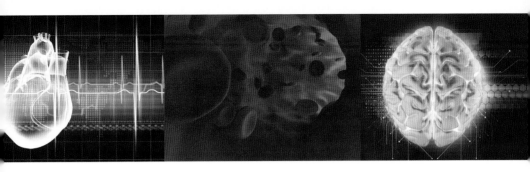

CHAPTER 10

Heart and Head

Cardiovascular disease (CVD) has many causes in people with and without diabetes. Risk factors include a family history of heart disease, high cholesterol levels, high blood pressure, cigarette smoking, obesity, inactivity, age, and the presence of albuminuria. Many of the risk factors can be controlled through lifestyle changes and medications **(Table 10.1)**.

Diabetes increases the risk of CVD. This association may be strongest in people with type 2 diabetes, who generally have metabolic syndrome, which includes overweight with fat carried mostly in the center of the body, elevated blood pressure, and low good cholesterol levels. These findings are not always found in people with type 1 diabetes, but most experts agree that there is an elevated risk of heart disease in people with type 1 diabetes.

While age is a risk factor for heart disease, the duration of type 1 diabetes is also a critical factor in assessing risk. A 30-year-old who has had type 1 diabetes for >20 years is likely to be at risk of CVD, while a recently diagnosed person of the same age would be at substantially less risk.

TABLE 10.1   Risk Factors for CVD

Risk factors that can be managed	Risk factors you can't control
High blood pressure	Age
Smoking	Sex
High blood cholesterol	Heredity (family health history)
Lack of regular activity	Race
Obesity or overweight	Previous stroke or heart attack
Diabetes	

Source: American Heart Association.

Heart Talk

The medical lingo related to heart disease can get a little confusing. Here is a rundown of a few important terms that tend to get confusing.

Macrovascular complications: Diabetes complications are often lumped into two groups: microvascular complications and macrovascular complications. The "micro" and "macro" prefixes refer to the tiny and the large blood vessels in the body, respectively. Large blood vessels feed the heart, brain, and limbs, so diabetes complications related to these body parts are included under the macrovascular umbrella. (We'll cover microvascular complications in the next chapter.)

Cardiovascular disease (CVD): Despite the "cardio" prefix, cardiovascular disease affects more than the heart. CVD is the medical term for a group of conditions predominantly related to the development of atherosclerosis, a buildup of plaque on the inner surfaces of the body's large blood vessels. CVD raises the risk of heart attacks and strokes. There are three major types of CVD most often associated with type 1 diabetes. These are blockages in the blood vessels of the heart (coronary artery disease), legs or arms [peripheral vascular disease (PVD)], and brain (cerebrovascular disease).

Cardiovascular event: A sudden blockage of blood flow to heart (heart attack) or brain (stroke).

Heart attack (myocardial infarction): A blockage that disrupts the flow of blood to the heart.

Stroke (cerebrovascular accident): A blockage that disrupts the flow of blood in the brain.

Heart disease: Another term for CVD, made confusing because it encompasses conditions that are not related directly to the blockage of a coronary artery by an atherosclerotic process. Hypertensive heart disease, congenital heart disease, and cardiomyopathies are other kinds of heart disease.

Coronary heart/artery disease: CVD caused by atherosclerosis in the coronary arteries, which are the main vessels providing oxygenated blood to the heart muscle.

Peripheral arterial disease: PVD caused by atherosclerosis, the hardening of the large blood vessels that supply the legs and arms. This condition can increase the risk of disability and amputation.

Cerebrovascular disease: CVD caused by atherosclerosis in the large blood vessels that supply the brain.

An "Event"

"I was diagnosed as being a type 1 diabetic when I was admitted to the UCLA emergency room after being assaulted at a walk-up teller in 1987.

In 2004 I had a heart event after eating a spicy dinner.

In the 17 years between being diagnosed as a type 1 insulin-dependent diabetic and needing bypass surgery, I was relatively healthy.

Before the event in 2004, I never exhibited any coronary issue. In the evening after a meal, I checked my blood sugar and noticed it was extremely elevated, well over 300 mg/dL. I started dosing more insulin to bring it down along with getting as much water into me to try to lower it. Several hours passed without much change. I decided to go to an emergency room because I was not seeing any lowering blood sugar and became concerned. In hindsight I should have called an ambulance. I assumed my situation was diabetes related and had nothing to do with my heart.

I arrived at the emergency room and they noticed I was extremely sweaty without any other symptom. They decided to start testing and realized I was having a cardiac event. During the testing they ran a circulatory test and discovered I had nearly 70% blockage.

UCLA termed my experience a cardiac event and not a heart attack. As a precaution the doctors put in a stent to improve blood flow and then get me started on medication.

The "plan" of trying a stent would take care of it; after a couple of minutes, they decided a CABG would be the best result. So I had a stent and then three bypasses performed. I was admitted to the hospital with a four-day stay.

In hindsight, diabetes is a very serious condition that can affect not only food processing, hydration, and so forth but also your blood pressure and circulation. Insulin is only a partial method of combating diabetes, but diet and exercise help keep the progression of the condition in check.

Weighing the effectiveness of getting a stent over a CABG is simple. Overall the CABG is a better solution to a blockage situation because it creates new pathways to assist the existing pathways. The hope is if you can reduce the blockages through medication, diet, and exercise, you may not need further heart surgery. By the way, currently it's been 13 years without complications. According to my cardiologist, I will not need further surgery for a long time, perhaps never."

—Keith Jahr, 57, has had type 1 diabetes since 1989.

Glucose

The landmark Diabetes Control and Complications Trial **(see page 23)** found that those in the intensive treatment group had a lower cardiovascular risk over 20 years than those who had been in the standard treatment group. Better blood glucose management over a long period of time lowers the risk of all diabetes complications, so keep at it.

Kidneys

Diabetic kidney disease has long been associated with an increased risk of heart disease in type 1 diabetes. High blood pressure, which can damage blood vessels in the kidneys as well as the heart, may play a role. Protein in the urine is a sign of an increased risk of a future heart attack or stroke. Get the recommended screenings for kidney disease and start treatment as needed to protect your kidneys, heart, and brain.

Insulin Resistance

Insulin resistance is usually associated with type 2 diabetes. In this condition, the body no longer processes insulin effectively, leading to high blood glucose levels.

Insulin resistance is closely related to obesity, which may be present in people with type 1 diabetes. Among adults with type 1 diabetes, just as we find in adults without diabetes, about 1/3 are normal weight, 1/3 are overweight, and 1/3 are obese. Children with type 1 diabetes are as likely to be overweight or obese as children without diabetes. The combination of type 1 diabetes and insulin resistance (metabolic syndrome with central obesity, hypertension, and abnormal lipid levels) is sometimes referred to as "double diabetes" and is related to an increased risk of CVD.

People with type 1 diabetes may be at increased risk for heart disease and stroke, but they also respond well to preventive measures to help lower their risk.

The Right Tests at the Right Time

Fasting Lipid Profile

This test measures the amount of certain lipids in the blood. It is done after 8–12 h without food or drink besides water. Do be sure to drink plenty of water before the blood test so you are not dehydrated—it is harder to draw blood on someone who is dehydrated.

There is controversy as to the need for fasting for blood tests. One of the issues for people who take insulin is the concern that blood glucose levels will fall too low while going to or waiting for blood to be drawn. If you/your child needs to drink juice or eat glucose tablets before the blood draw, it is fine. Pure carbohydrate does not have any fat in it, so it won't alter lipid levels. Carry simple carbohydrates with you when you go in for the test (as you should anyway) and some food to eat after the blood is drawn. Also, ask your health-care provider if you need to fast for the blood test. Sometimes the answer is no, which saves a step.

The test measures the levels of the following:

LDL cholesterol: Bad cholesterol. To remember, think of the letter "L": you want this number to be "low" because it's the "lousy" cholesterol. LDL cholesterol levels are a good indicator of risk, and there are cutoffs based on age and other risk factors to determine how high is "high."

HDL cholesterol: Good cholesterol. You want this number to be high. In contrast to LDL cholesterol, the higher your HDL cholesterol is, the lower your risk of heart disease.

Triglycerides: An excess of triglycerides in the blood can signal trouble. Often these levels are high because the blood glucose levels are high, and the triglyceride level returns to normal when blood glucose targets are reached. If triglyceride levels are very high (>1,000) they increase the risk of inflammation of the pancreas, known as pancreatitis. But this is rare in people with type 1 diabetes (as opposed to people with type 2 diabetes where it is more common).

See a summary of different tests in **Table 10.2**.

TABLE 10.2   Right Test, Right Time

What to check	How often	Adult goals	Pediatric goals
A1C (this target should be individualized, especially in older adults)	Every 3 months	<7% (in general, but higher if issues with hypoglycemia and/or heart disease)	<7.5%
Blood pressure	Every visit	<140/90 mmHg; ideally 130/80 mmHg with history of disease	Less than the 90th percentile for age, sex, and height; elevated blood pressure should be confirmed on 3 separate days
HDL cholesterol	Every visit	>40 mg/dL for men; >50 mg/dL for women	
LDL cholesterol	Every visit	Individualized	<100 mg/dL
Triglycerides	Every visit	<150 mg/dL	<90 mg/dL
Complete foot exam (all patients should have their feet inspected at every visit)	Yearly	Normal	Normal
Kidney function	Every year or as recommended Children: annual screening for albuminuria with a random spot urine sample for albumin-to-creatinine ratio should be considered once the child has had type 1 diabetes for 5 years; estimate glomerular filtration rate at initial evaluation and then based on age, diabetes duration, and treatment	Normal urinary albumin-to-creatinine ratio (<30 mg/g creatinine) and normal estimated glomerular filtration rate (>60 mL/min/1.73 m^2)	Normal urinary albumin-to-creatinine ratio (<30 mg/g creatinine)

> Not all people with type 1 diabetes are at the same risk for heart disease, so it is important to know your own numbers and treat as needed.

MACROVASCULAR DISEASE RISK ACROSS THE LIFE SPAN

Children

Children with type 1 can exhibit early markers of CVD, including atherosclerosis, blood vessel stiffness, and other risk factors. That's why screening for signs of heart disease is essential starting at a young age. However, most children do not actually develop heart disease—this happens as they age. But we want to start early to lower the risk.

The American Diabetes Association recommends a fasting lipid profile soon after a type 1 diagnosis in children, starting at the age of 10 years. If there is a family history of CVD, screening should start as early as 2 years. If levels are abnormal (LDL cholesterol ≥100 mg/dL), annual testing is recommended. If levels are normal, testing every 3–5 years is recommended until adulthood.

Measuring blood pressure is simple and noninvasive; it should be checked at each routine visit. What is "normal" depends on a child's age, sex, and height. Health-care providers have charts for this kind of thing. Children found to have systolic blood pressure or diastolic blood pressure greater than or equal to 90th percentile for age sex and height (high-normal) or greater than to equal to 95th percentile for age, sex, and height (hypertension) should have elevated blood pressure confirmed on 3 separate days.

If the blood pressure is found to be high and is persistent, the child must be assessed as to why. Based on the findings of the evaluation, treatment is started, which could include a combination of diet, exercise, and medication. Children should also be advised to not smoke.

Adults

In adults not taking statins, it is reasonable to obtain a lipid profile at the time of diabetes diagnosis, at an initial medical evaluation, and every 5 years thereafter, or more frequently if indicated. If you have a high risk of CVD, which includes having had type 1 diabetes for ≥20 years, treatment to lower cholesterol levels may be needed no matter what the actual numbers show. Not all people with type 1 diabetes are at the same risk, and there is no one-size-fits-all approach to the treatment of CVD risk in type 1 diabetes. That's why it is very important to discuss treatment with your health-care team.

Checking blood pressure and weight at each routine visit is also recommended. Blood pressure levels that are consistently high will need treatment and weight issues should be discussed in people who are overweight. All of these factors go into the mix of decreasing the risk of CVD and improving long-term health.

Possible Signals of a Heart Attack or Stroke

If you experience any of the symptoms below, report them to your provider. Severe or sudden onset of symptoms may indicate a heart attack. However, symptoms need not be severe to indicate a problem and may come and go. Women are less likely than men to experience chest pain during a heart attack.

Heart Attack

Chest pain (angina) or discomfort
Pain or soreness in back, neck, jaw, arm, or stomach
Shortness of breath
Sweating
Tiredness
Weakness
Palpitations
Rapid heartbeat
Weakness or dizziness/light-headedness
Nausea or vomiting
Anxiety

Stroke

Headache (extreme headache)
Numbness, weakness, or tingling on one side of the body
Confusion and trouble speaking, swallowing, or understanding
Problems with taste, smell, vision, or hearing
Dizziness or trouble walking

Treatment

Children

If high-normal blood pressure or abnormal lipid levels are detected in children or adolescents, the first step is to evaluate lifestyle and make smart changes. Weight management and regular physical activity are key, as is limiting dietary saturated fat. If risk factors don't improve within 3-6 months, it's time to try medication. The goal of treatment is blood pressure consistently less than the 90th percentile for age, sex, and height.

If hypertension is confirmed (systolic or diastolic blood pressure consistently equal to or higher than the 95th percentile for age, sex, and height), medication should be considered right away. Lifestyle changes should also be made.

An ACE inhibitor or angiotensin receptor blocker should be considered for the initial treatment of hypertension. Girls should receive reproductive counseling and should be using effective birth control because both of these classes of drugs can cause birth defects.

After the age of 10 years, the addition of a statin is suggested in patients who, despite medical nutrition therapy and lifestyle changes, continue to have LDL cholesterol >160 mg/dL or LDL cholesterol >130 mg/dL and one or more CVD risk factors. The goal of therapy is an LDL cholesterol <100 mg/dL. Short-term trials suggest that simvastatin, lovastatin, and pravastatin are safe for use in children and adolescents; however, symptoms of muscle breakdown (rhabdomyolysis), which can be a side effect of statins, should prompt a call to your health-care provider. None of the medications are safe during pregnancy, and therefore teenagers (and all women) of childbearing potential should be counseled about this risk.

Adults

Eating a healthy diet, getting enough exercise, quitting smoking, and losing weight, if necessary, are the primary strategies for preventing CVD. You will also want to intensively monitor and manage blood glucose, blood pressure, and lipids. In most cases, medication will be necessary to bring blood pressure and lipids under control.

The use of statins is well recognized as the first line of treatment for elevated cholesterol levels and a higher heart disease risk in everyone, with or without diabetes. A statin is recommended in everyone who has had a heart attack, stroke, or other vascular problem. For others who have not had an issue with CVD, the use of a statin is considered on a case-by-case basis, first looking at all the risk factors and making an assessment.

You can find CVD risk calculators online. Plug in age, sex, smoking history, etc., and the calculator spits out your risk. There is a bit of conflict as to whether these risk calculators are accurate, and they lump together all people with diabetes, type 1 and type 2, which may not be appropriate, but they still provide an idea of the 10-year risk of heart disease.

A big factor in the risk of CVD is age. As you get older, your cholesterol levels tend to increase, and other factors come into play. There is not a lot of information about treating people under the age of 40 years, and women of childbearing age should use effective birth control if taking a statin because it can cause harm to a developing baby. If you plan to stop using birth control, tell your doctor.

There is also not a lot of information as to the benefits of statin use in people aged >80 years. By then you have lived long enough to prove that CVD won't kill you at a young age. However, there still may be a benefit of lowering your cholesterol levels. Most of the research is on people at risk of heart disease aged 40–80 years, and that is where much of our information comes from. In general, it is important to have a conversation at least once a year with your health-care provider to be sure you are optimally reducing your risk of CVD.

Hypertension medications are effective at lowering blood pressure in type 1 diabetes. Multiple medications are often needed to reach the target blood pressure of 140/90 mmHg, though mixing ACE inhibitors and angiotensin receptor blockers (ARBs) is not recommended. Other blood pressure medications include thiazides, calcium channel blockers, and β-adrenergic blocking agents.

For people who've had a heart attack, stroke, blood vessel damage in the limbs, or other severe CVD episodes, aspirin treatment is typically recommended. In some high-risk individuals, low-dose aspirin may be an appropriate preventative therapy. Additionally, there are other medications to prevent blood from clotting that tend to be given if someone has had a heart attack, stroke, or a procedure such as a stent.

See **Table 10.3 and Table 10.4**.

TABLE 10.3 Medications

Medication	Use	Side effects
Statins Atorvastatin (Lipitor) Fluvastatin (Lescol) Lovastatin (Mevacor) Pitavastatin (Livalo) Pravastatin (Pravachol) Rosuvastatin (Crestor) Simvastatin (Zocor)	To lower bad cholesterol levels and reduce risk of CVD	Muscle aches and pains (less commonly, rhabdomyolysis), nausea, sometimes liver function abnormalities
PCSK9 inhibitors Evolocumab (Repatha) Alirocumab (Praluent)	Injectable, very powerful at lowering bad cholesterol level; reserved for people at high risk who can't take statins or in whom statins are not enough	Injection site reactions, allergic reactions, flu-like symptoms, runny nose and cough, muscle pain
ACE-I/ARBACE-I/ARB **ACE inhibitors** Benazepril Captopril Ealapril Fosiniopril Lisinopril Perindopril Quinapril Ramipril Trandolapril **ARBs** Candesartan Eprosartan Irbesartan Losartan Olmesartan Telmisartan Valsartan	To lower blood pressure, treat kidney disease, help the heart; preventing heart attack and stroke	The most common side effect of an ACE-I is a persistent cough; ACE-I and ARBs can both cause sudden fainting, low blood pressure, excessive potassium in blood, and possible angioedema (swelling of tongue, lips, hands or feet)
Aspirin (usually 81 mg taken daily)	To help prevent blood from clotting to prevent heart attacks and strokes	Bleeding ulcers, upset stomach, bruising, allergic reactions

TABLE 10.4 Other CVD-Modifying Meds

Medication	Use	Side effects
Ezetimibe (Zetia)	Lowers cholesterol by reducing absorption in the gut; reduces cholesterol levels by 10–15%; mild reduction in CVD risk	Back pain, chest pain, diarrhea, headache, joint and muscle pain, upper respiratory tract infection, tiredness
Fibric acid derivatives	Lowers triglyceride levels; minimal benefit on reducing CVD	Nausea, upset stomach, occasional diarrhea; potential risks when combined with statins include myositis and rhabdomyolysis; greater risk of kidney injury with the combination of gemfibrozil and statins
Bile acid resins: cholestyramine, colestipol, colesevelam	Lowers cholesterol by binding it in the gut; gives a small reduction in CVD risk but in type 2 diabetes may lower the blood glucose level a bit as well; no data in people with type 1 diabetes	Bloating, fullness, abdominal pain, constipation, gas, heartburn; must take many pills per day
Supplements: red rice yeast, berberine, other	Red rice yeast acts a bit like a statin, whereas others have different effects; most not proven to reduce CVD, although RRY may	Supplements are not regulated by the FDA so dose/purity may not be standardized; all pills can have side effects and supplements are no exception; tell your health-care provider if you are taking supplements so they can be followed

TESTING FOR AND TREATING HEART DISEASE

To understand CVD, you must realize that it is a diffuse disease. This means that if you have it, it involves most, if not all, of the blood vessels in your body. The ones that people think the most about are the blood vessels that fuel the heart, known as the coronary arteries. These arteries can become clogged, and when that happens, a person has a heart attack. It also turns out that some of the arteries are more important than others. The left main/left anterior descending arteries lead to the main part of the heart muscle. Clogs here can often cause death, and abnormalities here are sometimes called the "widow-maker."

Because of the seriousness of a heart attack, and the fact that CVD is the leading cause of death in the U.S., doctors want to lower the risk of dying from heart disease. But what is the best way to do this? Through risk-factor reduction—eating a healthy diet, exercising, not smoking, taking cholesterol-lowering medication, reducing blood pressure and blood glucose levels—everything we talk about in this chapter.

In terms of testing for heart disease, the American Diabetes Association and American Heart Association recommend that if you have symptoms of heart disease such as chest pain, left arm pain, shortness of breath, unexpected tiredness, or an abnormal resting EKG, you should have testing with a treadmill test or another form of cardiac scanning/testing. If you have a very strong family history of heart disease you should probably be tested as well.

Cardiologists may find areas in your coronary arteries that are narrowed, where blood flow is reduced, so they put stents (a tiny, wire mesh tube) into these areas to increase the blood flow. Stents are put into the heart during an angiogram, when a tube is threaded into your heart and dye is injected into the coronary arteries so they can be seen in detail. If there is a significant blockage, a stent can be placed. Putting in a stent will help reduce the symptoms you had—the chest pain or shortness of breath. So you will feel better. However, stents, in many cases, do not reduce the risk of a heart attack, because the plaque is located everywhere. Just because one part seems narrowed doesn't mean that is the area where a heart attack will happen. The plaque is all over. So we are back to healthy lifestyle as the best strategy against heart attacks. Also, when you have a stent, you have to take blood thinners, which can increase your risk of a stroke and other forms of bleeding.

There are times when stents really help. If you are having a heart attack and get a stent, it can reduce damage to your heart and help you recover from the heart attack. But the treatment that has the biggest benefit is surgery—known as coronary artery bypass grafting. This means that a surgeon takes a relatively healthy blood vessel and bypasses all of the diseased blood vessel so that normal blood flow through a healthy vessel is restored. Surgery sounds like a much bigger deal than a stent (it is), but it is also much more likely to help you live a longer and healthier life.

> There are many tests for heart disease, although not all have been proven to lower your risk of heart attack or stroke. Be sure to find out which tests are recommended and why, and how they will help your future.

Table 10.5 lists the tests that are recommended in various circumstances. Ask your providers for their advice. Evaluation and treatment should always be individualized. For example, in a 45-year-old woman who has had type 1 diabetes under good management since she was 20 years old, the guidelines say to start a statin. But what if she has no risk factors? No family history for heart disease.

TABLE 10.5   Tests to Detect Heart Disease

Test	What it is	Who should have it and how often	What it can show
EKG	A simple test to see if the heart has had certain types of damage	People at risk of heart disease, which is in general most people with diabetes; to be done every 1–2 years	Old or current damage to the heart
Coronary calcium scan	Low-dose CT scan	People for whom it is not clear whether treatment is needed for heart disease risk; done every 5 years if negative	Calcium in the coronary arteries, which is a sign of plaque buildup
Exercise treadmill test/nuclear treadmill test	Exercising on a treadmill to see what happens to the blood flow to the heart under stress	Anyone with symptoms of heart disease	A possible narrowing of the arteries in the heart that needs further testing
Pharmacologic stress test	Ways to stress/monitor the heart in people who can't exercise enough for the exercise treadmill	Anyone with symptoms of heart disease who can't do the regular exercise test	A possible narrowing of the arteries in the heart that needs further testing
Echocardiogram	An ultrasound of the heart	Anyone with a heart murmur or heart failure or other conditions that can alter the structure of the heart	Abnormal heart structure in terms of the valves and walls of the heart; how well the heart is pumping
Holter (or other) monitor	A patch or device that is worn for several days to continuously record the heartbeat	Anybody with abnormal heart beats, including rapid heart rate, irregular heartbeats, and other issues	Abnormal heart beats, including the heart beating too slowly or too quickly or irregular beats
Angiogram	Catheters (tubes) that are fed in through the veins to get to the arteries that feed the heart with blood; dye is injected to see if there are blockages	Usually done after one of the tests above is significantly abnormal	Severe blockages in the blood vessels around the heart that require either a stent or surgery to repair

She exercises and eats well, her blood pressure is completely normal, her weight is in a good range, and her good (HDL) cholesterol level is high (potentially protective). She has a low bad (LDL) cholesterol level, and she has no symptoms of heart disease. Does she really need a statin? How does she know?

One way to tell is with a coronary calcium scan. This is a simple, low-dose CT scan that shows whether there is calcium in the coronary arteries. Calcium means that there is cholesterol building up in the arteries. If there is no calcium present, it is a very good sign, and it may mean that medication is not needed. If calcium is present, more testing may be needed and starting a statin would be appropriate. If negative, the coronary calcium scan should be repeated every 5 years or so at the direction of your health-care provider.

Many other tests are possible—CT angiograms, MRIs, PET scans—but their true additional benefit in terms of diagnosing treatable heart disease is not known in general or in people with type 1 diabetes in particular. Many conditions involving the heart happen more frequently in people with diabetes overall, such as congestive heart failure and atrial fibrillation. These topics are beyond the scope of this book, particularly because there is little independent knowledge of these issues specifically in people with type 1 diabetes.

> There is no better way to prevent or treat your risk for heart disease than to have a healthy lifestyle, know your numbers, and take medications as recommended by your health care team.

Whenever any testing or procedure is recommended for you, be clear on the reasons why you are having it done. Ask if what is being done will help prolong your life in a meaningful way. Treating symptoms is important if you are having chest pain or shortness of breath. But if you have no symptoms and don't have severe disease, aggressively lowering your risk factors for heart disease may be the best and safest approach. Speak with your health-care team and choose what is best for you.

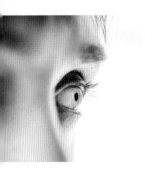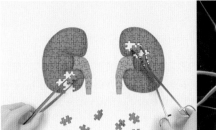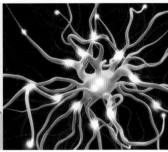

CHAPTER 11

Eyes, Kidneys, and Nerves

Tiny blood vessels permeate every corner of the body, carting nutrients to and waste products from cells. Type 1 diabetes can damage these delicate vessels, leading to microvascular complications: diabetic eye and kidney disease. Diabetic nerve disease shares some of the same risk factors and prevention strategies.

Scientists have learned a lot in recent years about how to prevent or slow the damage that leads to eye, kidney, and nerve disease in people with type 1 diabetes. With each passing decade, the risk of these complications in people with type 1 diabetes has declined.

DCCT proved that keeping blood glucose levels closer to normal levels lowers the risk of diabetic eye, kidney, and nerve disease. Other risk factors are beyond your control. The longer you've had type 1 diabetes, the greater the risk of these complications, regardless of blood glucose levels. Independent of duration, those who develop type 1 diabetes as children are more prone to complications than those diagnosed as adults. However, people who developed type 1 diabetes in childhood and are now aged ≥50 years did not have access to many of the new tools we have for treating diabetes. In the 1960s and 1970s, we didn't have self-monitoring of blood glucose levels. We don't yet know what complication rates will look like in children born during this current era of diabetes management and beyond. Certainly the opportunity for people to live long, complication-free lives has increased. Plus, some people with type 1 are lucky enough to continue to make tiny amounts of insulin, which may help delay the onset of complications. Finally, some people may be more prone to diabetes complications than others. We don't know how to determine this in advance, but there are some people who live long, complication-free lives with higher blood glucose levels. However, because we don't know who these relatively "protected" people are, everyone needs to try and keep their blood glucose levels as close to the normal range as possible.

> Remember, not every ailment that happens in a person with type 1 diabetes is due to diabetes. Sometimes a stomach ache is just a stomach ache, not a diabetic issue.

One important consideration when navigating health care is that, although type 1 diabetes is associated with a long list of possible complications, diabetes can't be blamed for every health issue. This is a common misconception among doctors. Stomachache? *It must be gastroparesis, a common type 1 diabetes complication.* But usually a stomachache is just a stomachache.

A child, adolescent, or young adult with type 1 diabetes may worry about diabetes–related complications occurring down the road. Educate your child in a positive way that emphasizes staying healthy and strong and taking care of diabetes so that these health problems can be prevented. Scaring a tween or teenager with the possibility of complications is not an effective way to motivate them to take better care of their diabetes. In fact, it often has the opposite effect.

EYES

If Someone Tells You...

"Like many people, I had the wake-up experience that changed everything. We had moved from the outskirts of Death Valley to a rural town on the eastern side of the Sierra Nevada Mountains, population 500. I was taking my adult community college class on a field trip to the Museum of Contemporary Art in Los Angeles. We had just started the 200-mile drive when I saw what turned out to be a bleed on the inside of my right eye. We completed the trip and a few days later I was able to make an appointment with a visiting ophthalmologist who came to a town 60 miles away from us once a month. The diagnosis was proliferative diabetic retinopathy.

I arranged to travel to the Reno, NV, area for laser treatment, having over 800 blasts in each eye per visit over several months. During one of these visits the doctor rather nonchalantly told me I would be blind within 5 years. Not a very big deal for him I guess. But kind of a big deal for me. I had already started seeing a new physician at the local clinic near where we lived. He was young and just out of his residency and working at a rural health clinic to help pay off his student loan obligations. I knew about the studies showing that tight control leads to fewer complications, and I knew I didn't have much control at all, let alone tight. The new doctor was fresh out of school and knew about the latest in diabetes management, including type 1. My A1C was 13. I started using mixed insulins of NPH and Regular and doing fingersticks multiple times a day and watching my diet more carefully. This was 1985 and fingersticks could be done with the new devices that used a spring-loaded needle, rather than a blade, and color-coded test strips.

If I was going to be blind, I had to start making some decisions about the future. My son was graduating from high school and my daughter had two years to go. I had been teaching part-time with emergency credentials and was planning on finishing up a teaching credential program because I really liked teaching. Being blind and teaching art, even ceramics and sculpture, would be a challenge.

With my new regimen, I felt great. The retinopathy was under control and I decided to go ahead with my plans while I could. When my daughter graduated, I went back to school full-time in the Los Angeles area and came home on the weekends. I contacted the American Diabetes Association for referrals for diabetes specialists and started seeing one regularly. He recommended an ophthalmologist who specialized in proliferative retinopathy. Big lesson: when someone tells you that you will be blind within 5 years, get a second opinion.

My new physician didn't know why the original doctor thought I would go blind. He had done a good job with the laser treatment, and I just needed a few touch-up treatments. My diabetes was well controlled. No new bleeds. And there were a lot of procedures that could be done to prevent blindness. Finished up my Single Subject Credential in Visual Art and went home to teach for another 25 years."

—Drew Wickman

At Diagnosis

People who have very high blood glucose levels at diagnosis often notice that their vision is blurry and "off." This happens because falling blood glucose levels change the shape of the lens—the glucose in the blood falls more rapidly that glucose in the eye. This is a temporary problem. It is not serious and generally goes away over about a month. People should see an eye doctor to be sure there is nothing else wrong, but in most cases there is not. Don't buy eyeglasses during this period because the eye tests will be off until the eye settles back down to normal.

Retinopathy

The major vision-threatening complication caused by diabetes is retinopathy. Your retinas are nourished by a system of fine blood vessels. Diabetes can damage these blood vessels, causing them to leak or rupture. If the damage is severe, vision can be lost. Serious changes caused by diabetes often cause no symptoms until it is too late. Fortunately, we now have many ways to help prevent the progression of retinopathy **(Fig. 11.1)**.

There are several forms of retinopathy.

> We have more ways than ever before to treat diabetic eye disease, and as long as people go in for their screening tests much blindness can be prevented.

Nonproliferative Retinopathy

By far the most common type of retinopathy, nonproliferative retinopathy occurs at some point in time in almost everyone who has had type 1 diabetes for long enough (although not always). There aren't any symptoms; only an eye doctor using specialized tests can detect the narrowed or blocked retinal blood vessels that define nonproliferative retinopathy. These are little red "spots" (little

A retina without any damage.

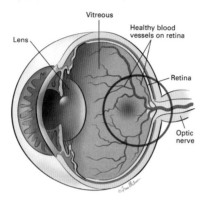

A retina with some diabetes damage.

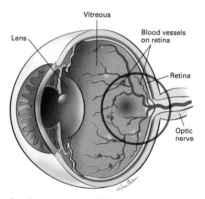

A retina with a lot of diabetes damage.

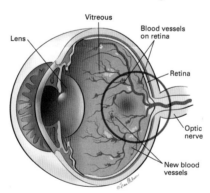

FIGURE 11.1   Diabetic eye disease can affect many parts of the eye, including the retina, macula, lens, and the optic nerve.

drops of blood) on the back of the eye. They don't cause loss of vision on their own and often can go away with tight blood glucose management. However, they are also a sign that some slight damage is occurring and that blood glucose goals should be reached and maintained over the long haul.

Macular Edema

Sometimes without warning, nonproliferative retinopathy can trigger macular edema. The macula is the central part of the retina. The accumulation of fluid or other substances from leaking blood vessels under the macula causes it to swell, which can distort vision, like a buckling mirror. Untreated this can lead to a loss of central vision. Often people may not know they have this, which is why annual visits to the eye doctor are a must for any person with any degree of diabetic eye damage.

Proliferative Retinopathy

If retinopathy moves into its second stage, it becomes proliferative retinopathy, which can threaten eyesight. When diabetes damages the retinal blood vessels, the body attempts to fix the situation by growing new blood vessels. Unfortunately, the plan can backfire. These new growths tend to be fragile and are prone to breakage and leaking. The leaking blood can cause spots in the visual field at first and may lead to blurred vision or worse as the leakage progresses. Some people are aware of their eye filling up with blood (on the inside). This can be frightening at first, but fortunately it is reversible in many cases. The blood may clear on its own or resolve as a result of treatment. Very rarely it continues to block eyesight.

Children: Children aged <10 years are mostly safe from retinopathy according to many experts; however, the risk goes up in adolescence. As many as 7% of adolescents who have had type 1 diabetes for only 2–5 years have early-stage retinopathy. After 5 years, the prevalence goes up, though sight-threatening eye disease remains rare in young people. In children, as in adults, the risk of retinopathy is related to blood glucose levels, with those who have the highest glucose levels at the greatest risk. Even though it is very uncommon to see retinopathy in children and adolescents, blood glucose management in early childhood and more so in adolescence is important and does impact the risk of developing retinopathy and other complications down the road.

Adults: Sometimes, an adult with very high blood glucose levels will decide to quickly get blood glucose levels to goal. This may happen around the time of wanting to have a baby or when a person with chronically high glucose levels simply decides to finally bring them down. In DCCT, we learned that this rapid change in blood glucose levels can make the back of the eyes look WORSE, not better. This can be very upsetting to the person with diabetes, but over time the abnormal changes in the eyes get better and overall eyesight worsens much more slowly because of the good management rather than continuing to get worse.

Cataracts, glaucoma, and other eye disorders are more common in people with type 1 diabetes than in the general population. In older adults, these eye problems become more common and can also cause changes in vision. Therefore, the challenges to keeping one's eyesight normal are greater. Additionally, if people have a loss of vision they may need special help when dealing with their diabetes care.

Get Screened

One of the greatest success stories in type 1 diabetes over the last few decades is the preservation of eyesight, which is due to better screening and blood glucose and blood pressure management as well as better treatments if eye disease happens.

In many countries, and in some places in the U.S., retinal cameras are used for screening for eye disease. These cameras take pictures of the back of the eye, and a person reading the photos can look for any changes. These cameras are helpful, but there are other types of eye disease that can be missed (like glaucoma), and the best test is probably a dilated examination by an eye-care specialist who is knowledgeable in treating people with diabetes. Your eye doctor will put drops into your eyes so the pupils become large and then take photos and make measurements to see if there is any swelling in the back of your eye and give a thorough examination. The gold-standard screening method is fundus photography, which can visualize the health of the retinal blood vessels.

Go see your eye doctor right away if you have symptoms of retinal detachment, such as seeing a new floater or flashes of light, having what seems like a veil over your vision, or any other changes in vision.

Children: The American Diabetes Association recommends that people with type 1 diabetes begin to get annual screenings for retinopathy from a trained professional starting at the age of 10 years or at the start of puberty (whichever occurs first) AND after they have had diabetes for 3–5 years. This means that a toddler with type 1 diabetes will not need their first retinopathy screening exam until they go into puberty or reach the age of 10 years, even if they have had diabetes for 8 years. Of course your child should have their age-appropriate vision screening done like children do without diabetes.

Once they reach the point of needing their first screening exam, this should be repeated every year or two depending on average blood glucose levels, age, and recommendation of the eye professional. Many parents ask if the eye professional should be an optometrist or ophthalmologist, and generally either is fine along as they have expertise in screening eyes for diabetes-related eye changes.

Adults: The American Diabetes Association recommends that people with type 1 diabetes begin to get annual screenings for retinopathy from a trained professional starting 5 years after diagnosis. The provider can also check for other eye conditions at this time. However, in many people with adult-onset type 1, which often progresses more slowly than type 1 in children, we don't know exactly when the blood glucose levels start to rise, so it may be wise for all adults to get their eyes checked when they are diagnosed.

In general these examinations should be done every year, but in people with no eye disease and very good blood glucose levels, the frequency may be switched to every other year. But as people age, so does their risk of all eye diseases. Adults may need more than one eye doctor—one who specializes in the front of the eye, for cataracts or glaucoma, and one who is an expert in the back of the eye (for changes caused by diabetes or macular degeneration).

Prevention

Keeping the eyes healthy boils down to two main factors: blood glucose and blood pressure. The evidence for the importance of blood glucose comes straight from the DCCT, which compared tight (goal A1C <7%) to standard management. Tight management lowered the risk of developing retinopathy by 76% over the long term. High blood pressure is linked to worsening retinopathy, though the bulk of this data comes from studies in type 2 diabetes. Still, maintaining healthy blood pressure levels (<140/90 mmHg in adults and <90th percentile for age, sex, and height in children) is a safe bet.

Treatment

Laser photocoagulation cuts severe vision loss and blindness by 90% in people with nonproliferative or proliferative retinopathy. Heat from the laser seals off or destroys the leaking, damaged blood vessels that contribute to vision loss. The laser can either be focused on a specific part of the eye, such as the macula, or scattered around the eye to target many problem blood vessels. Multiple treatments may be necessary to thoroughly eradicate problem vessels.

A newer retinopathy treatment involves injecting medication directly into the eye. The injection contains a drug that blocks the activity of vascular endothelial growth factor (VEGF). This hormone promotes the formation of new blood vessels and plays a key role in retinopathy by spurring the growth of weak, leaky blood vessels. Anti-VEGF drugs put a stop to problem vessels, improving vision in people with retinopathy. In many cases these treatments have to be repeated every few months (sometimes every month) to decrease the inflammation in the eye. Many people think of an injection into the eye as something horrible, but this is done quite gently, with local numbing medication, and most people don't mind it.

There are also some other new treatments, with substances that are put into the back of the eye to help it heal. All of these advances in eye care have made a big difference in helping people's eyes. Prevention is always first, but if damage happens, it can be treated.

KIDNEYS

The kidneys are the body's filters, letting waste pass through and into the urine for excretion while reabsorbing valuable nutrients into the blood **(Fig. 11.2)**. Diabetes can damage the kidney's tiny filters, leading to diabetic kidney disease (also known as nephropathy). Obviously this can be a very serious issue and at its worst can lead to dialysis or kidney transplantation. However, reducing rates of kidney failure in people with type 1 diabetes has been another big success in modern diabetes management. Because of better blood glucose AND blood pressure management, as well as newer medications, over 90% of people with type 1 diabetes will NOT develop serious kidney problems. This is an important lesson on the power of good diabetes care to prevent a major problem.

> Most (over 90%) of people with type 1 diabetes will never have any kidney damage, and good control of blood pressure and blood glucose levels will reduce the risk further.

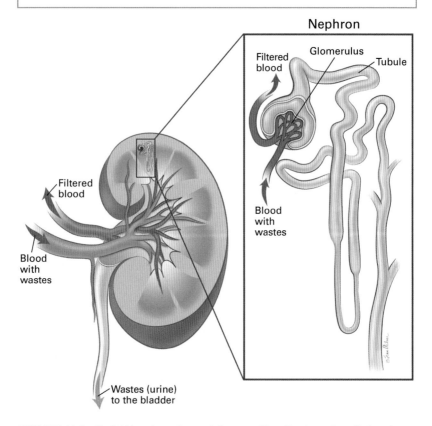

FIGURE 11.2   Each kidney is made up of about a million filtering units called nephrons.

Detecting Disease

When damaged, the kidney's filters become leaky. Health-care providers can detect leaks by checking the urine for the protein albumin, which is retained by healthy kidneys. Any increase in the urinary albumin is called albuminuria. Another window into kidney health is a blood test that looks for creatinine, a chemical waste byproduct associated with muscle metabolism. Healthy kidneys get rid of creatinine, no problem, but damaged kidneys can let some creatinine stick around the body. Creatinine levels can be translated into a glomerular filtration rate—a measure of how quickly your kidneys process waste (the glomerulus is the medical name for the structure in the kidneys that performs the filtering).

Albuminuria is often the first sign of diabetic kidney disease, followed by a decline in glomerular filtration rate. It is easy to test for kidney damage—the earliest signs can be seen on a urine test and later with a blood test.

Keep in mind that diabetes isn't the only cause of kidney disease. People with a family history of nondiabetic kidney disease, short duration of diabetes, a lack of other diabetes complications, impaired glomerular filtration rate without albuminuria, or other factors need to be evaluated for alternative explanations.

There are various stages of diabetes kidney disease, starting with the mildest form and progressing to the most serious, which is kidney failure. Fortunately, early kidney damage can be treated, preventing progression to more serious stages. **Table 11.1** describes the stages of kidney disease. The stages of chronic kidney disease are based on a combination of information from both blood and urine tests. You should ask your health-care provider for the results of your kidney function tests when you have it measured each year.

TABLE 11.1   Stages of Chronic Kidney Disease

GFR stages	eGFR (mL/min/1.73 m²)	Terms
Stage 1 (or G1)	>90	Normal or high
Stage 2 (or G2)	60–89	Mildly decreased
Stage 3a (or G3a)	45–59	Mildly to moderately decreased
Stage 3b (or G3b)	30–44	Moderately to severely decreased
Stage 4 (or G4)	15–29	Severely decreased
Stage 5 (or G5)	<15	Kidney failure

Albuminuria stages	AER (mg/d)	Terms
A1	<30	Normal
A2	30–300	Moderately increased
A3	>300	Severely increased

A GFR is calculated from a blood test and is a measure of how well your kidneys are working. AER, albumin excretion rate; GFR, glomerular filtration rate.

Children

Children should have a urine test for albumin starting 5 years after the diagnosis of diabetes. While albuminuria is detected in ~15% of adolescents, in most cases, the elevated urinary albumin resolves on its own. Even if it persists, kidney function is rarely compromised in children and adolescents with type 1 diabetes. For these reasons, medications for kidney disease are rarely prescribed for those aged <18 years. If a child or adolescent develops protein in the urine and has had relatively short duration of diabetes with reasonable glucose management, it is important that nondiabetes-related causes of the protein be evaluated and ruled out.

Adults

An annual urine test for albuminuria starting 5 years after diagnosis with type 1 diabetes is also recommended for adults, plus a serum creatinine test at least annually. However, in adults this urine test is often done at diagnosis, much like the eye exam, because it is hard to know how long an adult with type 1 diabetes has actually had high glucose levels. Also, adults may have high blood pressure, which increases the risk of kidney damage.

Management

While there aren't kidney-specific medications, blood pressure medications can prevent or delay the development of diabetic nephropathy **(see Table 10.2)**. For patients without albuminuria, any of the four classes of blood pressure medications (ACE inhibitors, angiotensin receptor blockers, thiazide-like diuretics, or dihydropyridine calcium channel blockers) that have shown beneficial cardiovascular outcomes may be used. Often more than one blood pressure medication is needed, since it is particularly important to keep the blood pressure levels down. ACE inhibitors and ARBs should not be taken during pregnancy. Women of reproductive age should use effective birth control if taking them and should talk to their doctors about having their blood pressure medications adjusted when pregnancy is planned, before stopping birth control.

> High blood glucose levels can damage nearly every nerve in the body; preventing permanent nerve damage is a very good reason for keeping blood glucose levels in the normal range.

NERVE DAMAGE (NEUROPATHY)

Researchers don't entirely understand how diabetes damages nerves. There's more to it than high blood glucose levels, but the details are fuzzy. Neuropathy is common in people with type 1 diabetes, especially if blood glucose levels are high for many years. Rates go up in those who've had diabetes longer. Children can also show signs of nerve damage, though it's often asymptomatic; symptoms tend to emerge at older ages. High blood glucose levels, elevated triglycerides, excess weight, smoking, and high blood pressure are risk factors for neuropathy.

There are many different types of diabetes-related neuropathies. The most common, peripheral neuropathy, affects the nerves in the hands, feet, legs, and arms. It generally starts in the feet, and it tends to start in both feet at once. This condition manifests with a variety of symptoms, including numbness, tingling, pain, weakness, and a loss of motor skills or balance. Often the symptoms, especially those of burning or shooting pain, are worse at night. Eventually the painful symptoms stop and the patient is left with a chronic feeling of numbness or coldness in their feet.

Rarely a sudden, severe form of neuropathy can occur, which we think is caused by loss of blood flow to one specific nerve. For example, this can happen to the nerves that control one eye or the nerves that go to one side of the abdomen or thigh. These mononeuropathies (meaning one nerve) will come on quickly but also go away fairly rapidly (over weeks to months).

Another common form of neuropathy is autonomic neuropathy, which can contribute to heart, bladder, and gastrointestinal conditions, as well as erectile dysfunction. This can also cause variation in blood pressure: blood pressure can fall too low upon standing and lead to dizziness or lightheadedness (orthostatic hypotension).

Sometimes having a high blood glucose level can make nerves tingle or cause some dizziness. Athletes may develop a subtle form of orthostatic neuropathy if their glucose levels are too high and may require more electrolyte-containing fluids than other athletes to keep going. These symptoms do not mean that there is permanent damage but rather a good reminder to keep blood glucose levels in the normal range.

There is another much more serious but VERY rare type of nerve damage that comes from sudden correction of extremely high blood glucose levels—in the range of 300–500 mg/dL—maintained over several years. These patients, often young adults, will decide to get their blood glucose levels into goal range, begin giving adequate amounts of insulin for the first time in years, and quickly reduce their glucose levels down to the normal range—close to 100 mg/dL. This sudden fall in blood glucose levels causes sudden damage to the nerves in the feet and legs. The pain these patients experience is very severe. It may be partially reversible but does not entirely go away.

The way to prevent this is to slowly improve blood glucose levels in people who have been chronically high for many years. This is different from people with new-onset diabetes, who have not experienced high glucose levels for years. A more gradual reduction in blood glucose levels also helps reduce some of the weight gain that can happen if insulin is introduced too rapidly.

A variety of tests can be used to detect the different types of diabetic neuropathies. Treatment is a challenge, but strategies to minimize pain and improve function are available. The right test and treatment depends on the type of neuropathy. In general we cannot reverse or "cure" nerve damage, so it is very important to prevent it by keeping blood glucose levels in the normal range.

Peripheral Neuropathy

Real Pain

"My neuropathy has grown from my feet to my ankles to my calves. The pain has steadily been increasing over the year and has gotten to the point where it has changed my lifestyle. I work a good portion of the day from bed so I can keep my legs up. I have had to abandon my business traveling.

Last night we met a fantastic artist, a fascinating older woman. She paints and writes plays. We were standing as we visited her. It was after walking around for over an hour. I told her we needed to go because my ankles were killing me and the bottom of my feet felt like they were burning up.

It feels as if parts of me are slowly dying. The ankles are real pain. At times they feel as though they are swollen although they don't appear to be. One Sunday, I had a nice creative day sitting in my bar stool at the kitchen counter. That night when we got into bed I looked at my feet and they were swollen. You could not see the veins or bones. My feet look like they belong to an alien creature. I spent all day Monday in bed and by Tuesday the swelling had subsided. Since then I make sure I don't sit too long or stand. I really don't expect there to be any magic pill for me. But on the off chance there is something, I'd gladly give it a try."

—Eric Lichtbach, 61, has been executive director of a
family manufacturing company since he was 19.

While keeping blood glucose levels in goal range can prevent peripheral neuropathy and keep it from getting worse, there aren't any treatments that can reverse nerve disease once it's established. Once neuropathy is detected, the focus is on keeping the feet and legs healthy and on managing pain.

Pain Management

Several medications are cleared for use in the treatment of pain from diabetic neuropathy. The first-line therapies are anticonvulsants and antidepressants, followed by opioids. While effective, opioids are lower on the list because their use can lead to substance abuse. They're typically reserved for when other treatments fail. Some topical agents, such as nitrate sprays and capsaicin, may also reduce pain.

Foot Care

If you have nerve damage and can't feel the bottoms of your feet, you won't know if you get a small cut or sore on your foot. Pain is a signal that something is wrong. If there is no signal from the nerves, you need to use your eyes to see if there is something amiss. Otherwise you may keep walking on an irritated part of your foot and make it worse. It may seem simple to say, "Look at your feet every day," but often people don't do this as a matter of habit, and some older people may have trouble with arthritis or vision and have difficult actually seeing their feet.

In addition to nerve damage, people with diabetes may also have problems with their circulation. A loss of blood flow slows healing. Finally, high blood glucose levels make it hard for wounds to heal. Together, nerve and blood vessel damage with high blood glucose levels cause nonhealing foot wounds called ulcers, which increase the risk of amputation. However, all of this can be prevented by looking at your feet.

Adults: Annual screening for peripheral neuropathy is recommended for all adults with type 1 diabetes starting 5 years after diagnosis. There are several standard screening tests that assess sensation in the foot. For example, your health-care provider will see if you can feel the light touch of a filament or sense the vibration of a tuning fork. Again, diabetes isn't always the culprit behind a loss of sensation; alcohol abuse, renal failure, thyroid disease, genetics, and vitamin B12 deficiency can also trigger neurological damage. These causes must be ruled out before diabetes is implicated.

The use of specialized therapeutic footwear is recommended for those with severe neuropathy, foot deformities, or history of amputation. People with neuropathy or evidence of increased plantar pressures may need only well-fitted walking shoes or athletic shoes that cushion the feet and redistribute pressure. People with bony deformities (e.g., hammertoes, prominent metatarsal heads, bunions) may need extra-wide or extra-deep shoes. Some people with bony

---

Foot Patrol

During a daily foot check, look for these signs of trouble. If you spot any of the symptoms in this list, see your health-care provider or podiatrist promptly to prevent problems from getting worse. These concerns are primarily for people with "high-risk" feet: those with nerve or blood vessel damage or past foot ulcer amputation. Although checking one's feet is never a bad idea, it is most important if the foot is already damaged.

- A change in the size or shape of the foot
- A change in skin color (becoming red or blue)
- A change in skin temperature (warmer or cooler)
- An open area of skin (blister or sore) with or without drainage
- An ingrown toenail
- Changes in structural deformities of the foot (hammer toes or bunions)
- Changes in corns or calluses

deformities, including Charcot foot, will need custom-molded shoes. Medicare and other insurances will often help pay for needed footwear.

Children: Many parents are told that their child shouldn't play outside with bare feet, that they can't wear flip flops, and that they should check their child's feet regularly. Children with diabetes have feet like children without diabetes, so we recommend that parents use common sense. Children with diabetes have normal sensation and circulation in their feet and should have normal wound healing if they were to get a scrape or cut. Proper toenail care is important to prevent ingrown toenails, however. Your diabetes care provider is unlikely to screen for neuropathy in the feet until the child is a teenager and has had diabetes for longer than 5 years, although they may want to check that the toenails are being properly cared for.

AUTONOMIC NEUROPATHIES AND MORE

Since nerves stretch throughout the body, damage manifests in a wide variety of forms.

Cardiac Autonomic Neuropathy

Damage to the nerves that regulate heart rate can lead to cardiac autonomic neuropathy (CAN), which increases the risk of CVD. There are many systems that regulate heartbeat and function, and for most people these work well. But an occasional person will have what is known as orthostatic hypotension, which means that your body can't adjust to a change in position from lying down to sitting or standing. Although we rarely think about it, when you change positions your body has to figure out how to continuously send blood to your brain and other organs. When you are flat, this is fairly simple. But when you stand up all of your blood vessels need to squeeze a little bit tighter to keep the blood flowing upwards. This adjustment happens because your autonomic nervous system tells your blood vessels to react. If this doesn't happen, you can feel lightheaded or dizzy when you sit or stand up. This has happened to nearly everyone at one time or another in their lives, but if orthostatic hypotension develops, this happens nearly every time the person changes position. The test for this is to have your blood pressure tested when you go from sitting to standing—healthy people's blood pressure increases upon standing, while those with CAN have a hard time regulating blood pressure. There are other causes of this besides diabetes, so be sure to let your provider know if you have these symptoms. There are also many ways to treat it.

Gastroparesis

Nerves orchestrate the flow of food through the digestive tract. Damage to the vagus nerve, which controls the passage of food through the stomach, can lead to a diabetes complication called gastroparesis.

Tips for Healthy Toes

- Check feet daily for signs of trouble.
- Get annual comprehensive foot exams to identify risk factors for ulcers and amputations. In addition, your health-care provider should inspect your feet at every visit.
- Outfit the feet in supportive shoes in the correct size and moisture-wicking socks. If you wear high heels, be sure they fit well and check for any pressure spots or blisters.
- Contact your health-care provider if you notice anything abnormal.
- Remember that if you have no nerve damage or decrease in blood flow and your glucose levels are well managed, your feet are much the same as everyone else's. But be sure to be a little extra protective of your feet.

Tips for People with Neuropathy

- Remember that your eyes are the key to sensing foot problems; the nerves to your feet will not give warning signals, so look at your feet every day.
- Check the bottoms of your feet whenever you put on shoes or take them off.
- If needed, set a mirror on the floor to see your feet.
- See a podiatrist as often as recommended, especially if your toenails are abnormally thick and need cutting by a professional.
- Have your health-care provider check your feet at EVERY visit.
- Either wear orthopedic shoes designed for your feet or check with your provider(s) to be sure your shoes are appropriate.
- Keep shoes, socks, and feet clean and dry.
- Avoid wearing shoes with elevated heels. Because of nerve damage, you may have poor balance and be at risk of falling.
- Contact your podiatrist or other health-care provider ASAP for any changes in your feet, including challenges staying balanced.
- Don't smoke! (That applies to everyone.)
- Have the blood flow in your feet checked every year by your health-care provider.
- Exercise as tolerated and allowed by your health-care team.

Wildly fluctuating blood glucose levels may be one sign of gastroparesis. For example, if food remains in the stomach for longer than is typical, the insulin taken before a meal will hit the bloodstream before the glucose from the food does, leading blood glucose levels to go low. Then later, once the food is finally digested, the insulin has left the body, so the glucose from the meal remains in the circulation, leading to blood glucose highs. Other symptoms of gastroparesis include nausea, vomiting, reflux, feelings of fullness, bloating, and abdominal pain or discomfort.

Gastrointestinal (GI) symptoms happen commonly, and only rarely is gastroparesis the cause, at least with modern diabetes management. But if it is a concern, get tested for gastroparesis. You'll eat or drink food that is labeled with radioactivity, and then the amount of time it takes to go through the GI tract is measured. Having a high blood glucose level itself can slow gastric emptying, so this test should be done once blood glucose levels are better managed, or at least below 200 mg/dL at the start of the test. Often patients with any sort of GI symptom are told they have gastroparesis. However, on testing MOST don't. People with diabetes can get the same GI problems as nondiabetic people, although in addition to gastroparesis, it is important to rule out celiac disease.

Some treatments for gastroparesis are behavioral: eating smaller meals and fibrous well-cooked foods can improve symptoms. Medications and "pacemakers" that stimulate the stomach muscles may also be prescribed. Using an insulin pump may make it easier to balance insulin dosing with food absorption, particularly using such features as dual or combination boluses, or extended bolus dosing.

Charcot Foot

This is a type of neuropathy that leads to a breakdown of the bones in the foot. Often, at first, the foot is red and warm and looks infected, but it isn't. In general it happens because of many different problems—nerve damage with loss of sensation, autonomic nerve damage, high blood glucose levels, injury to the foot, inflammation, and abnormal bone structure. The foot seems to almost collapse, often losing the arch of the foot. This is called a "rocker" bottom foot and can lead to problems with balance and mobility. Treatment may include immobilization, efforts to reduce swelling, and medications that improve bone structure. With better diabetes care, this is becoming less common but needs to be recognized immediately if it happens so that medical treatment can be given.

Bone and Joint Issues

On a cellular scale, bones are constantly being broken down and built up again. Type 1 diabetes can get in the way of this cycle, leading to a range of bone and joint conditions, including such conditions as frozen shoulder. The tendons that allow the hands to flex and move can also undergo various changes due to diabetes, leading to carpal tunnel syndrome, trigger finger (stenosing tenosynovitis), limited joint mobility, and Dupuytren's disease (contracture). Stiffness or limited mobility in the hands are symptoms of these conditions. There is something called the "preacher sign" that is common in people who have had type 1 diabetes for a long period of time **(Fig. 11.3)**. Some of these conditions can be treated by medications or simple surgeries. Unfortunately, improving blood glucose management does not improve these abnormalities. Testing for diabetes complications is crucial and should be done on schedules recommended by your diabetes team **(Table 11.2)**.

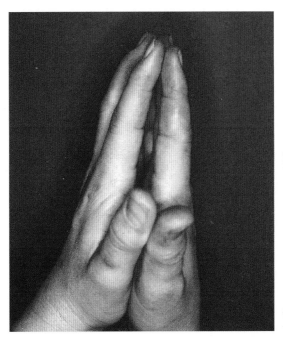

FIGURE 11.3   Preacher sign of stiffness and limited mobility. The person is not able to bring the palms together.

Source: Bolognia JL. Skin and subcutaneous tissues. In *Therapy for Diabetes Mellitus and Related Disorders*, 5th edition. Lebovitz HE, Ed. Alexandria, VA, American Diabetes Association, 2009, p. 436.

TABLE 11.2   Testing Schedule for Diabetes Complications

	Test	Starting	Frequency
Eyes	Dilated eye exam	5 years after diagnosis (and ≥10 years old)	Yearly
Kidneys	Urine test for albumin Blood test for creatinine	5 years after diagnosis	Yearly (or more)
Nerves	Foot exam	5 years after diagnosis (and ≥10 years old)	Yearly

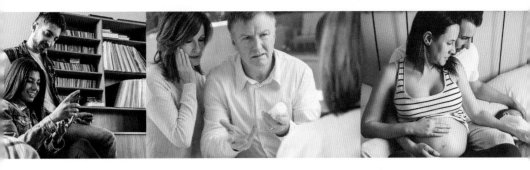

Chapter 12

Sexual Health for Him and Her, and Reproduction

With all the other health topics to discuss at the doctor's office, it's easy to let concerns about sexual issues slide, since it can be an uncomfortable subject to broach. But silence is a mistake.

Your health-care provider can offer suggestions or prescriptions to improve specific sexual problems. Just as important is that sexual dysfunction can be a warning sign of other health problems. This makes sense because many types of diabetes-related sexual dysfunction stem from blood vessel damage, the same underlying cause of heart, eye, kidney, and nerve complications.

His

Sexual dysfunction in men takes three common forms: erectile dysfunction, problems achieving orgasm, and low libido (sex drive).

Diabetes-related nerve damage may cause erectile dysfunction. However, it's important to check for low testosterone levels (hypogonadism) before sticking diabetes with the blame.

If testosterone levels are low then it can be replaced, but this isn't as simple as it sounds. If you want to father a child, then you shouldn't take testosterone—it stops the production of normal sperm and can take months to years to recover from. In older men, testosterone can increase the red blood cell count, which may increase the risk of heart attack and stroke. Some of the oral anabolic steroids can cause liver damage. So testosterone is a hormone that should only be taken after a discussion with a health-care provider about its pros and cons, and follow-up blood tests are necessary.

If the problem is primarily erectile dysfunction, certain medications, such as Viagra, Levitra, and Cialis, are known as PDE5 inhibitors and work well. Ask your doctor if one of these is right for you. If you still have difficulty, see a urologist, who can discuss the range of options with you and choose the treatment plan that works for you.

Emotionally Painful

"I have traveled the world, built a business, been loved and in love with some wonderful women in my lifetime. I'm finally having to live with some of the effects of having diabetes for 42 years.

When my sweetheart has romantic interest, I can't make any performance promises. It's nothing to laugh at. When you love someone, you want to give them everything you possibly can. Not to be able to provide that special gift that puts a click in her heels and gives her a reason to keep you around and put up with all your boy stuff, like tools in the kitchen, is emotionally painful. But I remind myself that any day you can put your own clothes on and feed yourself is a great day. All in all, I have lived a great life."

—Eric Lichtbach

Hers

When it comes to puberty, periods, sex, and pregnancy with diabetes, it is all about being prepared and knowing how to get ready. When you/your child are entering a new phase in life, speak to your health-care provider.

About a third of women with type 1 diabetes from the DCCT reported sexual problems, including loss of libido; problems with orgasm, lubrication, and arousal; and pain. Depression is a big risk factor for sexual dysfunction. Treating depression may help improve the sex lives of women with type 1. Unfortunately, some antidepressants can reduce sex drive even as they reduce depression. Strategies that may improve your sex life include the use of lubricants and assistance from a sexual health professional, who may have ideas for how to address this issue.

Practical Matters

Just like any other form of physical activity, when you have sex your glucose level can drop and it can keep dropping afterwards. As with other types of activity, it is helpful to be prepared to prevent low blood glucose.

- Check blood glucose before and after sex—a particularly vigorous session could cause a dip in blood glucose.
- Adjust insulin or eat a snack if needed.
- Have a glucose source handy.
- Tell your partner that you have diabetes.
- If you use an insulin pump, it may be safest to disconnect before having sex to avoid infusion set entanglements.

DIABETES AND PREGNANCY

Women with type 1 diabetes can have successful and healthy pregnancies, but the importance of planning cannot be stressed enough.

Before Conception

Type 1 diabetes increases the risks for birth defects, including microcephaly, miscarriage, and preterm delivery. However, these risks are greatly reduced if you achieve blood glucose goals for pregnancy—an A1C of <6.5% or as close to normal as possible without excessive hypoglycemia—*before* conception. In other words, the best outcomes for healthy moms and healthy babies are achieved if blood glucose goals are reached before the pregnancy even begins.

Birth Control

Use effective birth control until *1*) you want to have a baby and *2*) blood glucose levels are in the target ranges. Conversations about sexual activity and pregnancy prevention need to start in the early teenage years with your child's pediatrician, family doctor, or endocrinologist.

There are multiple forms of effective contraception, from oral medication to intrauterine devices and contraceptive implants. Choice of birth control should be decided with your health-care team. In general the options are similar to a woman without diabetes, although occasionally hormonal forms of birth control may cause increases in blood glucose levels and insulin doses will need to be adjusted.

Be Prepared

When you decide you want to get pregnant, but before you stop using birth control, tell your health-care provider. You will need to meet at least monthly to establish tight blood glucose management, make a nutrition plan, and address additional health issues that may complicate pregnancy. Generally this requires a team, including a diabetologist, a registered dietitian, a CDE (often a nurse or nurse practitioner), and an obstetrician. Be sure to find an OB who is used to treating a person with type 1 diabetes—many treat women with gestational diabetes, but this is very different than treating someone with pre-pregnancy type 1 diabetes. Additionally, you should have a retinal exam performed by your eye care provider to be sure your eyes are in good shape for pregnancy (see details below).

It's a good idea for both you and your partner to meet at least some subset of the diabetes team. Pregnancy is a challenge on its own; add it to type 1 diabetes and the complexity increases. You will need a support system both before and after the baby is born. Your partner should be ready to give glucagon if you have a severe low blood glucose reaction. Your partner can also help with shopping and meal preparation to be sure mother and developing baby have the right food choices for a healthy pregnancy.

The Dreaded Third

"I'm at the end of my second pregnancy with type 1 diabetes. It took me a long time to get comfortable with the idea of being pregnant with type 1. I didn't have the confi-

dence that I could do what it takes to have a healthy baby. I was really worried that high blood sugars would cause harm to my baby, and for this reason my husband and I seriously considered surrogacy (even asking his sister to carry for us after we met with fertility doctors).

Not really having a great surrogate option plus having some really reassuring conversations with other type 1 mommas, I decided to go for it. It is a lot of work, but to my surprise was definitely doable! My A1Cs were in the 6s and 5s for the first time in my life! Diabetes definitely took front stage in my life. I altered the way I ate, worked, traveled, exercised, and followed up with my diabetes team.

My first pregnancy was very stressful. I had just moved to a new state and started a new job, so life was anything but routine. Also, with every high blood sugar, I worried that I was harming my baby. Every ultrasound brought a sigh of relief. The heart anatomy ultrasound came back normal (sigh.) The limbs were forming normally (sigh). The baby was moving and growing (sigh).

The good thing is you get to see your baby A LOT as a type 1! In the third trimester, I went to my high-risk OB's office two times a week for monitoring. I gave birth to a healthy baby boy at 38 6/7 weeks via planned C-section, no NICU time, no low blood sugars for me.

My second pregnancy came quickly after my first. This pregnancy has been harder in some ways, and easier in others. It's hard to give diabetes the focus it had during my first pregnancy because I am taking care of my toddler. That being said, I have the confidence to know that I can do what needs to be done. My blood sugars have been a little easier to control this time. I'm in the middle of the dreaded third-trimester insulin resistance. It's harder to prevent those post-meal high blood sugars and even harder to bring those blood sugars down. Interestingly, 160 is high for me now. Nonpregnant I would never say that!

The biggest difference for me being pregnant vs. not being pregnant is the attention and effort. I carb count, log meals, send in data to my team regularly, see my endocrinologist more often, see my diabetes educator more often, etc. It all pays off, though."

—Natalie H. Strand

Blood Glucose Management

Ideally, you'll reach the A1C target of <6.5% before you get pregnant. This shifts to a target of <6% during pregnancy. Sounds impossible? It isn't. Even women with high and erratic blood glucose levels can reach and maintain these targets before and during pregnancy. In a way the harder part is after pregnancy, when life is complicated by the presence of a baby. Too often women revert to their old habits, with a higher A1C. This is understandable but not desirable because it is good management over a lifetime that leads to long-term health with type 1 diabetes **(Table 12.1)**.

Sometimes A1Cs <7% can be achieved with daily periods of high blood glucose levels. Blood glucose crosses the placenta into the baby's circulation and triggers the baby's pancreas to secrete extra insulin. These high glucose levels in the baby can create a lifelong abnormality in terms of how they respond to the food environment. So when planning pregnancy, it is important to keep those

TABLE 12.1   ADA-Recommended Targets During Pregnancy

Fasting	≤95 mg/dL
1 hour after eating	≤140 mg/dL
2 hours after eating	≤120 mg/dL
A1C	A target of 6–6.5% is recommended, but <6% may be optimal as pregnancy progresses

These values represent optimal levels if they can be achieved safely. In practice, it may be challenging for women with type 1 diabetes to achieve these targets without hypoglycemia, particularly women with a history of recurrent hypoglycemia or hypoglycemia unawareness. Hypoglycemia may increase the risk of low birth weight.

spikes down as well as reduce the A1C. If your A1C is close to target and your blood glucose levels, based on monitoring, are all excellent, your diabetes care team may consider you ready to conceive even if the A1C doesn't quite reflect all of the improvement just yet.

A flexible insulin plan—multiple daily injections or an insulin pump—is recommended during pregnancy. Both are equally effective in pregnancy; however, some providers prefer pumps. At the end of the day, it's a personal decision. If you are going to switch to an insulin pump, do so well before you go off birth control.

Some insulins are Category C (risk to fetus not ruled out), so your doctor may have you switch to a different insulin.

Nutrition during Pregnancy

Meet with a CDE and a registered dietitian to review carbohydrate counting, dining out, and incorporating snacks as needed. If needed, losing excess weight before pregnancy can reduce the risk of a range of obesity-related pregnancy complications. Be consistent with meal and snack times to help smooth out the peaks and dips in blood glucose levels. Take folic acid supplements to reduce the risk of birth defects, and make sure you are getting enough calcium and vitamin D.

Diabetes Complications and Pregnancy

Pregnancy will put your body under significant stress. If you have diabetes complications or are at increased risk, you may need to take extra care when planning for a pregnancy. However, with most complications, mother and baby will be fine. It is simply important to be aware of any areas of particular concern.

Kidneys and Pregnancy

Kidney disease is detected by measuring urine levels of a protein called albumin. Preeclampsia, a pregnancy complication, is detected in the same way. It's helpful to know the status of your kidneys going into pregnancy so doctors know what is going on. If you develop protein in your urine due to pregnancy, it should go away after pregnancy, as it does in a woman who does not have diabetes.

If you have some degree of kidney damage, speak with a kidney specialist (nephrologist) before you get pregnant. Maintaining a normal blood pressure during your pregnancy will be particularly important.

There are some very rare cases when you could be told that your kidneys are not healthy enough to tolerate a pregnancy. If that happens, discuss options with your health-care team. There are women who have had kidney transplants (and therefore have normal kidney function) and have gone on to have successful pregnancies. The key to success here, as it is with all aspects of pregnancy, is to plan and prepare thoroughly.

Eyes and Pregnancy

One study found that 10% of women without retinopathy developed the condition during pregnancy; in over half of those with preexisting retinopathy, it got worse during pregnancy. Women with high blood glucose levels, rapidly improving glycemic levels, longer diabetes duration, hypertension, and preexisting retinopathy are at increased risk of worsening eye health during pregnancy. Even so, pregnancy itself is NOT a risk factor for retinopathy over the long-term, so it is likely the pregnancy-related retinopathy will not be permanent, so long as other risk factors are kept in check. This serves as an important reminder that as a woman is considering pregnancy, she should work with her medical team to ensure that her diabetes is very well managed 3 months before and throughout the pregnancy to maximize her health and the health of her baby.

Have your eyes checked before you get pregnant. If you have no eye disease, then you will likely need to be checked only during the first trimester. If you are found to have active eye disease needing treatment, you will need treatment before conception, because some of the treatments for eye disease (injections into the eyes) can't be given once you are pregnant. A concern would be progression of untreated proliferative retinopathy during pregnancy, for which laser might have been chosen prior to conception.

Finally, as with kidney disease, there are rare cases when a woman has such serious eye disease that she can't risk becoming pregnant without going blind. This happens much less often these days now that we have such good treatment for diabetic eye disease, but it is important to know if this is a risk.

Blood Pressure and Pregnancy

Getting blood pressure to target is another health issue to take care of prior to pregnancy. In a pregnancy complicated by diabetes and chronic hypertension, target goals for systolic blood pressure 120–160 mmHg and diastolic blood pressure 80–105 mmHg are reasonable. Unfortunately, the hypertension medications often used for people with diabetes—ACE inhibitors and ARBs **(see page 124)**—are not recommended during pregnancy because their use is associated with birth defects. Tell your doctor that you are planning to go off birth control so that your medications can be changed safely. There are other medication options that are safe for pregnancy, and these should be started before conception to be sure they are effective.

Heart Disease and Pregnancy

If you are older and have had type 1 diabetes for >20 years, ask your health-care provider to be sure you don't have heart disease prior to planning a pregnancy. If you have heart disease, discuss the possibility of pregnancy with a cardiologist. Women with certain kinds of heart disease can die during pregnancy.

Autoimmune Diseases and Pregnancy

Thyroid disease, celiac disease, and other autoimmune diseases are more common in people with type 1 diabetes than in those without the disease. Screening for these conditions is recommended in the pregnancy-planning stages, as these diseases could be harmful to a pregnancy and would need management.

Pregnancy

Growing fetuses get their nutrients from mom's blood. This includes glucose, which can fluctuate widely in women with type 1 diabetes. High maternal blood glucose levels can cause excessive growth in the developing baby and can have a lasting impact, increasing the risk of obesity and insulin resistance in chil-

---

Preconception Checklist

Ready to take the plunge into parenthood? Here's how to get ready:

- Get your A1C below 6.5% and as close to normal as possible without hyperglycemia or significant hypoglycemia.
- Take a folic acid supplement daily (600 mg).
- Talk to a registered dietitian who is familiar with diabetes and pregnancy.
- Get an eye exam to check for retinopathy.
- If retinopathy is detected, get treatment before conception.
- Have your kidneys checked out with urine (albumin-to-creatinine ratio) and blood (serum creatinine) tests.
- Get a thyroid function test.
- If you have risk factors for heart disease (see Chapter 10), talk to your doctor about screening for heart disease.
- Tell your health-care provider that you are planning to go off birth control and follow instructions about changing any of your medications.
- Consider bringing your partner with you to an appointment with your diabetes specialist. He/she may have questions to ask, and it may help to review the use of glucagon because the risk of severe hypoglycemia increases with tighter control.

---

dren and adolescents. This is why tight blood glucose management is very important leading up to and during pregnancy. Low blood glucose levels, however, do not generally cause harm to the fetus, even though they can be disruptive to the mother.

Insulin and Blood Glucose

Early in pregnancy, the body tends to be more responsive (sensitive) to insulin and later in pregnancy it become less sensitive (more resistant) to insulin. Your total daily insulin dose may change weekly throughout your pregnancy **(Table 12.2)**.

Avoiding DKA **(see page 85)** during pregnancy is critical for fetal health. DKA can actually occur at lower glucose levels than is typical. Pay close attention to glucose levels and measure ketones if your glucose levels stay above your target for more than a few hours and don't respond to correction doses of insulin that you and your medical team have previously discussed. Contact your health-care team if your ketones are positive or you are concerned. If you cannot fix the situation at home, getting intravenous fluids, with or without intravenous insulin, usually quickly fixes the problem.

Hypoglycemia

It's hard not to overshoot when striving to get blood glucose down to as close to normal as possible. It is not unusual for some pregnant women with type 1 diabetes to develop hypoglycemia with a blood glucose <50 mg/dL on 1 out of every 5 days, with as many as 70% experiencing severe hypoglycemia—blood glucose low that requires help from another person—at least once during pregnancy. The risk seems to be highest during the first trimester. This may be linked to the morning sickness and nausea that is common during this stage of pregnancy, although it also happens in women without morning sickness. A bit of good news: blood glucose lows don't directly increase the risk of birth defects or fetal death.

Consume carbohydrates at consistent times during the first trimester and be sure you are well equipped with appropriate snacks to treat hypoglycemia: glucose tabs, glucose gels, candies, etc. It is okay to give glucagon in pregnancy. Have your partner review how to give glucagon and practice with an expired kit.

TABLE 12.2   Insulin Needs during Pregnancy

Pregnancy stage	Insulin needs
0–9 weeks	Increase
9–16 weeks	Decrease
16 weeks	Low
16–37 weeks	Double or more
37–40 weeks	May decrease
Immediately after birth	May drop to half of prepregnancy doses

Hypoglycemia-induced dizziness, confusion, or loss of consciousness can cause car accidents, so, as usual, check your blood glucose level before getting behind the wheel. And more generally, checking blood glucose frequently is the best way to prevent and rapidly treat mild cases of hypoglycemia, and hopefully prevent severe hypoglycemia. Some women check as many as 10–20 times throughout the day and night during pregnancy. Continuous blood glucose monitoring, with its low glucose alarms, may be helpful during this more challenging time.

Complications
Thyroid
Up to a third of women with type 1 diabetes have Hashimoto's disease, an auto-immune disorder of the thyroid. The thyroid plays an important role in pregnancy, and thyroid disease can lead to pregnancy complications and birth defects.

Get checked for thyroid disease before you become pregnant. If thyroid hormone levels are low, they can be replaced with pregnancy-safe medications to restore healthy hormone levels. Your dose may need to be increased during the first trimester of pregnancy. Be sure your health-care provider follows your thyroid hormone level every trimester and adjusts your medications appropriately.

Women without existing thyroid disease can develop postpartum thyroiditis: thyroid hormone levels increase after delivery and then fall to low levels. If you are feeling nervous, sweaty, or shaky, are losing weight too quickly or having palpitations (fast heartbeat) in the several months after delivery, have your thyroid hormone levels checked.

Depression
An estimated 10% of women experience depression during pregnancy. The number is higher in women with type 1 diabetes and can negatively affect health of mother and baby. Certain antidepressants can be safely taken during pregnancy. Discuss this with your health-care provider if you are taking these medications before pregnancy or if you become depressed during pregnancy.

Hello, Baby
Delivery
In the past, many women with type 1 diabetes had C-sections due to concerns about diabetes causing a high-risk situation. With experienced obstetricians, more women with diabetes are going to term with their pregnancies and having vaginal deliveries. Follow the recommendations of your OB, and make sure that you are monitored and safe in the weeks leading up to delivery.

During labor and delivery, intravenous insulin is generally started and continued throughout the process. Sometimes the pump is left on and the doses managed in conjunction with the labor and delivery staff. Institutions have varying policies and procedures for the delivery process and it helps to learn what these are in advance. In the weeks leading up to delivery, your endocrinologist might create a plan for you to follow immediately after your baby is born. Regardless, bring all your diabetes supplies to the hospital so that they are available if needed.

After your baby is born and the placenta is removed, there is an immediate drop in insulin resistance. You will become very sensitive to the action of insulin. Generally insulin is held until blood glucose levels start to rise, usually within the first 24 h after delivery. Know what your pre-pregnancy insulin doses were and start back on a dose that is ≥10% below baseline levels. Key to management is, as always, adjusting based on blood glucose levels.

Not So Alone

"Although it was definitely hard, keeping my A1C under 6 wasn't the hardest part of my pregnancies. It was having to be induced simply because I was a type 1 diabetic. I wanted my babies to come out when they were ready, not because 'it's protocol.'

My 2-year-old son asks me where his medicine is every time he watches me take insulin via syringe. I tell him hopefully he will never have to worry about that. But to humor him, I give him an empty insulin vial. He clutches it in his hand around the house. And for some reason, it makes me feel like I'm not so alone."

—Amirah Meghani

Breast-Feeding

Breast-feeding helps mom drop excess weight, improves infant bonding, and lowers the child's future risks of obesity and type 2 diabetes, among other benefits. Plus, it saves you money! The American Academy of Pediatrics recommends exclusive breast-feeding for 6 months, followed by at least another 6 months of breast-feeding plus supplemental feedings. There is some, slight, data that avoiding exposure to cow's milk for the first year may reduce the risk of the development of type 1 diabetes in a child. Therefore, many women avoid feeding cow milk or cow milk–based products for the first year.

Women with type 1 have a few extra challenges when it comes to breast-feeding. C-section rates are higher in women with diabetes, which can make it more difficult to initiate breast-feeding. Infants of moms with type 1 are more likely to have latching issues. And women with type 1 may make less milk than is necessary to completely satisfy a child, requiring supplementation. Finally, there's the issue of hypoglycemia: expelling carbohydrates into breast milk can increase your risk of blood glucose lows.

These barriers are mostly manageable with the help of an experienced lactation consultant. One of the best ways to get into the habit of breast-feeding is to stay with the infant after birth—encouraging skin-to-skin contact and nighttime feedings.

You'll need a new pattern of giving insulin to account for breast-feeding and new patterns of being up at night. Generally, this is relatively easy to adjust for since moms are by now so used to having well-managed diabetes.

If you are not going to breast-feed, consult with your pediatrician as to the best source of formula for your child. You don't need to feel like you are short-changing your baby if breast-feeding doesn't work out. It has certain advantages, but you, with support from your medical team and key family members, will make the best choices for you and your child.

Thyroid disease can affect milk production, but the medication that's used to replace the missing thyroid hormone is FDA-approved for use during breast-feeding. Some medications for preventing heart disease and treating depression may pose risks to a breast-feeding infant. Discuss any medications you are taking with your pediatrician.

Birth Control

You can become pregnant soon after having a baby. In the weeks leading up to delivery, discuss your birth control options with your OB.

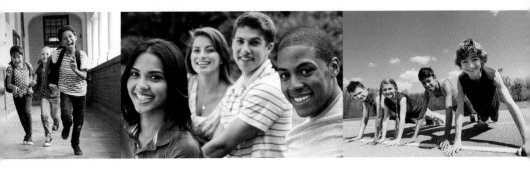

CHAPTER 13

Preteens, Teens, and Young Adults

As children grow up, they begin to separate from their parents. This is a normal part of development. But when a child with a chronic condition grows up, they need to become increasingly responsible for their own self-care. This can be quite difficult for someone with type 1 diabetes, particularly if the disease started young and the parents are used to managing all aspects of diabetes care. Additionally, adolescence is a time of rebellion and change, which makes careful diabetes management difficult. It's no wonder that from the ages of 16–25 years the average A1C level is higher than at any other point in life.

There are four main themes to helping a young person transition successfully.

1. Start early (at age 10–12, depending on the child) to educate your child on the responsibilities of diabetes self-management.
2. Work with your child's diabetes care team to allow your child to gradually gain independence with diabetes care tasks while still being available to guide your child.
3. Find an expert in type 1 diabetes management for adults so there are no gaps in care.
4. Make sure that all details are organized and prepared so that the transition from the pediatric to adult doctor occurs easily.

> Teens and young adults tend to have the highest blood glucose levels of any group; however, in general they transition to adulthood with much improved control

TRANSITIONING PHASES

Age 10–13

The age range of 10–13 years is often referred to as the "tween" years. Children of this age have usually mastered the developmental challenges of middle childhood. They have achieved "self-efficacy," which is the knowledge of what to do and the ability to do it. Most tweens this age can check their own glucose levels, have an understanding of how to treat a low or high glucose, can count carbs, and can give their own injection or bolus on an insulin pump.

However, there is a spectrum, and each child masters these skills at a different rate. And that is okay. Some 10-year-olds are very independent. There are 13-year-olds who still need help calculating the dose and are not independently bolusing or giving injections. Where kids are in this spectrum depends on maturity level, how long the child has had diabetes, their desire for independence, and their parents' comfort level in letting them become independent.

Even if a tween has the ability to do diabetes-related care tasks independently, he or she still needs close supervision by an adult. A confident and independent 13-year-old with diabetes may be able to manage their own diabetes day-to-day without a lot of adult supervision, but they shouldn't have to. This is a huge burden and can often contribute to diabetes burnout.

Tweens tend to still be "rule followers" and rise to the challenge of responsibilities and chores. They are gaining independence in other areas of their life: remembering to brush their teeth, bathe, get their schoolwork done, and keep their room picked up. You should allow your child to gain more independence with their diabetes as well. Allow them to stay after school with some friends, check a glucose on their own, and cover a snack with insulin. This is a gradual process and the parent or adult still needs to double-check that it went well.

Puberty makes blood glucose management more difficult, even if the tween and the parents are doing everything "correctly."

This early adolescent period is characterized by rapid growth and sexual maturation. In one word: puberty. This makes blood glucose management more difficult even if the tween and the parents are doing everything "correctly." Hormonal changes that are causing rapid growth and pubertal changes also cause insulin resistance, which results in higher insulin requirements. Emotional changes that come with puberty and more complicated peer relationships can also affect glucose levels. Insulin doses may need to be adjusted frequently; call your diabetes team for guidance if needed. Tweens, especially girls, who go through puberty and have their growth spurts earlier than boys, can sometimes need insulin dose adjustments every couple of weeks. Therefore, even if your tween is fairly independent with their diabetes care, stay involved enough that you know when glucose levels are heading out of range and adjustments are necessary.

Diabetes visits during this age range are still usually with the pediatric diabetes team. Expect your health-care provider to discuss growth and puberty with you and your tween, so that everybody has reasonable expectations and understands why diabetes is getting harder to manage. This is also the age when the diabetes team will be starting to screen for diabetes-related complications, such as retinopathy (eye problems), nephropathy (kidney problems), and cholesterol issues. These are rare in the tween years but this is when screening starts, especially if glucose levels were often high in the past or the tween has had diabetes for 5–10 years. This screening can make you and your tween worried. Remember—and tell your tween—that these tests are for prevention and are part of staying healthy and strong. Puberty is also a time for conversations about sexual activity and pregnancy prevention.

Time spent with the certified diabetes educator should be focused on transferring the diabetes knowledge from you to your child. The education should be more focused on the tween so that they gradually are learning everything that you learned over the preceding years.

> Teens want to be independent, yet still need some supervision and parental involvement with their diabetes care.

Age 13–18

Let us start out by saying that we love teenagers and they are a wonderful age group to work with. But teens often struggle with their diabetes management and this is the age range when we start seeing the A1C rise. Teenagers have a lot to master in all aspects of life, and adding diabetes into the mix is challenging.

By the end of the teen years, the young adult is supposed to have abstract thinking, be able to consider future implications and consequences of their choices, and be able to comprehend the impact of behavior on their future health. But this is easier said than done because teens are also risk takers, like to explore new behaviors, and tend to underestimate the negative consequences of their actions because they feel invincible. The challenge is that most teenagers do not fully develop these skills until their 20s. Teens want so badly to be independent with everything, including their diabetes, but they still need some supervision and parental involvement with their diabetes care. This desire for independence but continued need for parental involvement often leads to increased conflict around diabetes care tasks.

So how do we help the teen transition? We give them independence, but we stay involved enough so that we know when they need us to step back in. Two steps forward and one step back.

The teenager needs time alone with their diabetes provider so that they have the time to discuss the sensitive topics of relationships, sex, drugs and alcohol, and driving responsibilities. All education needs to be directed at the teenager, especially if they were diagnosed at a young age. The topic of transfer to an adult diabetes provider needs to be discussed years before it will likely happen so that there is ample time to plan, prepare, and gradually transfer diabetes care tasks to the young adult.

As they get closer to leaving home, the adolescent needs to be involved in scheduling appointments, ordering their medications from the pharmacy, dealing with sick days, and trouble-shooting on their own. Many pediatric centers offer courses and groups to help adolescents learn about transitioning their care, and these resources should be sought.

Emerging Adulthood

The age range of 18–30 years is considered the period of "emerging adulthood." In the old days people were married in their early 20s and started families; these days young people in their 20s are delaying this process with respect to marriage, parenting, and work. A theorist named J. J. Arnett has suggested that the post-adolescent period should be subdivided into an early phase corresponding to the years immediately after high school (~18–24 years) and a later phase when more traditional adult roles are assumed (~25–30 years).

In terms of the A1C, it seems that after reaching a peak in the late teens/early 20s, the A1C falls to the lower adult levels at around age 25 (**Fig. 13.1**). This can be encouraging to parents of transitioning youth—by the mid-20s, people become more capable of doing the diabetes self-management needed to have blood glucose levels in goal range. As a father of a young adult with type 1 diabetes puts it: "Keep them alive until they're 25." It turns out that brain development isn't finished until age 25, and the frontal cortex, the part of the brain involved with the most integrated, complex thought, is the last part to finish

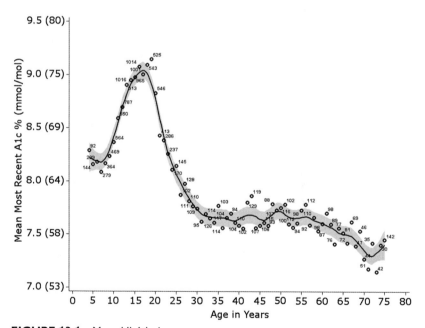

FIGURE 13.1 Mean HbA1c by age.

Source: Miller KM. Current state of type 1 diabetes treatment in the U.S.: updated data from the T1D Exchange Clinic Registry. *Diabetes Care* 2015;38:971–978.

myelinating (myelination is the production of the sheath that lines the nerve cells so they function normally).

> The more an adolescent can learn to do before they make the break from home, the easier the transition process.

During the early phase of emerging adulthood, the person may be moving away from home, attending school, learning how to support themselves, and separating from their parents emotionally. Competing academic, economic, and social priorities often detract from a focused commitment to diabetes management. Many young people don't feel adequately prepared to take on all of their own diabetes management, although in our experience the more an adolescent can learn to do before they make the break from home, the easier the process. Parents need to realize that a child, on their own, may be able to do more than they let on. But no matter how prepared the young adult is for the transition away from home, it is still a big change, in many ways.

The Worst Date

"Dating with diabetes—it sounds like a catchy soap opera title. Living in South Africa, I've become very fond of soapies, since most households watch them religiously. I can see it now!

Script: Samantha sits down next to the dashing young Thomas at her engagement party. She doesn't look well… 'Tom!' she squeals, 'I … I …' Her voice breaks. 'I need … glucose!' And promptly faints into her glittering plate of caviar and crackers.

The couple of dates I've been on, I've tried different methods of introducing my affiliation with needles and constant carb counting. I've even tested one potential partner's gag reflex by pulling out my needles without forewarning (not a very successful date tactic, it turns out).

One of the most difficult things about dating with diabetes is that some people are ignorant of how desperate the situation becomes when blood sugars go low. The worst date that I've been on, the person that took me out casually asked if I was going to finish my juice when I was low and whether it was possible if he could finish it! Despite staring at him in disbelief until he felt awkward, I learned from this experience to remember that I have had 23 very intimate years of living with diabetes. This first outing was, most likely for them, the closest to type 1 diabetes they have ever been."

—Mallory Bernstein, 24, is a Fulbright scholar and current
master's degree candidate at the University College London.
She has had type 1 diabetes since 17 months of age.

During the second phase of the young adult period, the 25- to 30-year-old often has a growing sense of identity and begins to enter into more stable, adult-like intimate relationships and full-time employment. During this time, people become more able to appreciate the importance of maintaining better blood glucose management to maintain health over the long term.

Life partners can be important supports. Bring new significant others to visits. The provider can answer questions and set the stage for how it is best to help—a balance between ignoring the diabetes and being the "diabetes police." Women will want to discuss contraception and targets for preconception and pregnancy.

Confidence and Courage

"After graduating college, just over two years from being diagnosed, I started working as an investment banking analyst at a major global financial institution. I wanted to prove to myself that I could manage diabetes and succeed in one of the most stressful job environments there is for a college graduate, working long hours, having to meet tough deadlines, and often having to manage ridiculous expectations from bosses. Perhaps without diabetes, I would have never had the drive and courage to pursue a career like this. And for that I have T1D to thank, knowing that I am successfully managing this disease has given me confidence and courage, has increased my-self-esteem, and has also often served as an ego check to remind me that I am human when I feel unstoppable."

—Jose Harari Uziel, 24, lives in Mexico City and works in investment banking.

THE TRANSITION FROM PEDIATRIC TO ADULT DIABETES CARE

> Adult medical care differs in many ways from pediatric care, which is something each transitioning youth needs to be prepared for.

One of the underappreciated issues in the transition from pediatric to adult care is how different the two models are for treating people with diabetes. Pediatric care is about families and interactions between the person with diabetes and their caregivers. If something goes wrong, it is the parent who is responsible.

The minute a person turns 18, all of the responsibility for health is now on the young adult's shoulders. Parents can only be included in the conversation if permission is granted. Sometimes transitioning young adults forbid providers from speaking to their parents, and this is a request the provider must honor.

There are basic differences in how diabetes care is given to pediatric and adult patients. Diabetes care for children requires involvement of the family in order to be successful. Young children do not have the ability to master diabetes management and teens often do not possess the emotional maturity to sustain the tasks of daily therapy. Although health-care delivery varies, in the pediatric health-care setting visits tend to be family-focused, holistic, and centered on management approaches that fit diabetes into the child and family's lifestyle. Diabetes visits and management approaches include parents/guardians as well as the youth.

In adult care, the focus is more on the independently functioning individual patient, who can be informed or counseled but then is expected to make his or her own choices about behavior or treatments. Adult visits tend to be substantially shorter and focused on medical problems. Adult patients choose who they do and do not want to have access to their health information and are largely considered independent consumers of health care. Whereas individuals change gradually from childhood to adulthood, the change in health-care provider can be abrupt and unsettling.

Another big difference is the other patients who go to see an adult endocrinologist. The people in the waiting room will not only be adults, many will be seniors. Type 2 diabetes is the more common form of diabetes, and even in an endocrinologist's office these are the patients most commonly seen. For younger individuals with type 1 diabetes used to a kid-friendly environment, this can be a bit of a jolt. Moreover, the office staff will expect the young adult to fill out any paperwork, show a copy of their insurance card and driver's license, and pay any co-pays and fees. There are no cartoon-themed stickers in an adult doctor's office.

Finally, many patients these days have to work hard to make the system work for them. It means planning ahead—asking for refills and insulin well in advance, having backup insulin (and long-acting insulin if on a pump), making sure glucagon is unexpired and urine ketone test strips are available. If a medication requires prior authorization from the doctor's office, this can take extra time, so be ready to wait. Appointments can be hard to schedule and should also be made in advance. If you miss an appointment and don't call to cancel 24 h or more in advance, you might be required to pay a fee. If you arrive late, you might not be seen. Young adults finally see how much their parents were doing for them with regard to coordinating the pieces of their diabetes care.

How to Make a Smooth Transition

In addition to preparing the child to assume responsibility for their own care, many steps can be taken prior to the transition. Parents, pediatrician, and the person with diabetes should all be involved. First, it is important to maintain health insurance coverage. Some can be covered on their parent's plan until age 26. If the parent lacks private health insurance, this transition in coverage will need to be made with the help of resources at the pediatric or new adult center for care, which may mean involving a social worker or a case worker.

Then there is the issue of when the transition should occur. For some it is easiest to stay with their pediatrician through college and then find a new provider when they settle in a new city. In general, diabetes visits can occur at school breaks and via phone/email. For others they may stay in the same city and need to switch providers because of insurance or programmatic issues. Others will want to switch to a new diabetes provider where they go to school or relocate. What is done depends on what the person with diabetes wants, what their insurance allows, and what is recommended by the pediatric team. When the transition occurs, it is often useful for the pediatric provider to create a letter or fill out a form that explains what has happened in the past. Examples of this form are available on various websites, such as the American Association of Diabetes Educators (www.DiabetesEducator.org). This information is often best transmitted in person—given to the young adult to be handed to the new health-care provider so that there is no delay.

When you are planning to go off to college, it helps to spend a visit or two going through all of the details of what it means to re-establish care in another location. This includes how to deal with local and mail order pharmacies. You will need to connect with student health; you may need to sign basic disability paperwork so that there is accommodation for tests or assignments postponed due to a diabetes-related issues. Check out CollegeDiabetesNetwork.org and their checklists for the months and weeks before you arrive.

Discuss how to safely approach drinking alcohol, and the effects recreational drugs and athletic-performance–enhancing drugs might have on diabetes management. Discuss your options for birth control.

Identify people who could help out in the event of an emergency. Have a plan if there are any problems. Many college campuses have a van that will pick up sick students and take them to student health. Find out which resources exist before they are needed.

One of the biggest problems for transitioning youth is getting "lost to follow-up," which means there is a gap in care. This happens far too commonly and when it does, not surprisingly, people do worse. Make use of the resources offered by your pediatrician to ensure that a connection is made with an adult provider before pediatric care ends.

> Young adults must never get "lost to follow-up." It is very important to always have a connection with a health care provider who can help you manage your diabetes.

The Bottom Line

Transition plans must start in the pediatric setting, years before they will actually occur. Ideally there will always be the "right fit" in an adult endocrinologist waiting to care for the young adult patient. However, endocrinologists are in short supply, and it may not always be possible to immediately connect with your adult "diabetes dream team" right off the bat. But young adults can and must continue to receive medical care in some fashion or another.

The key to making a successful transition is having a plan and the support to make it happen. Each person with type 1 diabetes needs at least one health-care provider who can write prescriptions for insulin and diabetes-related supplies. In a pinch this can be a primary care provider, a free clinic, or student health center.

The young adults who get lost in transition, who don't connect to new providers after leaving pediatric care, do the worst. By the time of the last visit in pediatric care, a new place for care should be clearly identified and an appointment set up. Concrete plans need to be made and followed. Understandably there are many competing issues as young adults grow up and leave home, but having diabetes necessitates a little extra planning and connection.

Choices exist as to which health-care provider you see. Young adults are often accustomed to simply following their parents in terms of who is the best doctor to followup with, but as an adult this is a more personal decision. If you see an endocrinologist with whom you don't feel comfortable or who doesn't answer your questions, shop around until you find one you like. This is especially true if you are settling into a place where you will live for a while. Ask for a recommendation from your pediatric provider before moving (and try to have an appointment planned and on the books for when you arrive), but you can also contact the local American Diabetes Association or JDRF chapters for information. In some health-care settings, you will need to find a primary care provider first to refer you to an endocrinologist. As long as the first connection with a provider is made, you should be safe and able to connect to the help you need.

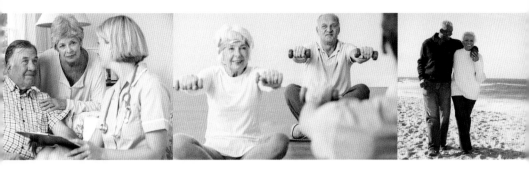

CHAPTER 14

The Golden Years

Type 1 diabetes is sometimes, mistakenly, thought of as a childhood disease. But the disease can show up in adulthood (it is estimated that half of all new-onset cases develop after the age of 20). People with type 1 are living longer, healthier lives than ever before, meaning we've got a robust population of older adults with type 1 diabetes.

Some older adults with type 1 diabetes are running races, while others reside in nursing homes. The key to living well into old age with type 1 diabetes, regardless of the specifics of your situation, is to make sure you're receiving personalized care that meets you where you are.

> Make sure all your health-care providers and family members know what type of diabetes you have and how to treat it. Too often, all older individuals are assumed to have type 2 diabetes and thus are treated inappropriately for type 1 diabetes.

Diabetes Type Confusion

A problem you may encounter in getting good care is that health-care professionals who don't know you may assume you have type 2 diabetes, particularly if you "fit the profile."

"William," an 80-year-old African-American man, experienced age-related confusion. When he went into the ER after a fall or for some other reason, the ER docs would stop his insulin, telling him he didn't need it because he had type 2 diabetes. Several days later he would show up in the diabetes clinic on oral agents with blood glucose levels in the 400–500 mg/dL range. He was just "following doctor's orders."

If you are overweight, you may be given unwanted advice by friends—or strangers—about how "diabetes can be cured, if you'd just eat right and lose weight." Having a simple sentence or two prepared to respond to "helpful" people can be useful.

Make sure all your health-care providers, caregivers, and family members know what type of diabetes you have and how to treat it. They need to know that if you don't get insulin, you can become seriously ill within hours. This information should be in your electronic medical record and recorded on smartphone health information apps. Wear a medical ID that says "Type 1 Diabetes—Insulin." Having an insulin pump can signal that someone has type 1 diabetes, but people with type 2 diabetes can also have insulin pumps, so it is often best to spell this information out clearly.

Long-Duration Diabetes

The risk of developing complications of diabetes increases over time. People living today who have had type 1 diabetes for 35 or more years were treated before we had tools such as self-monitoring of blood glucose, newer insulins, sensors, and modern pumps. It was much harder to keep blood glucose levels in the normal range and more common to develop some of the complications of diabetes.

The Joslin Medalist Study includes people with type 1 who've had the disease 50 or more years **(Fig. 14.1a and b)**. It's unclear if data from this study is broadly applicable, as these folks may represent an uber-healthy population of people with type 1, but the findings are interesting nonetheless. Some participants have had no significant complications from their diabetes and are living active, healthy lives. And given the fact that outcomes for people with type 1 diabetes are improving with improved treatments, it is hoped that people who live long lives with type 1 diabetes will have even fewer complications in the future.

(a) 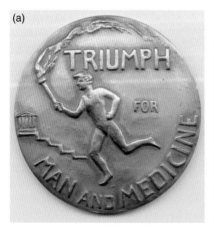 (b)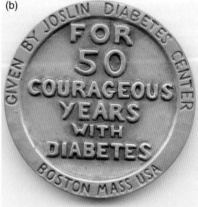

FIGURE 14.1 The Medalist Program at Joslin Diabetes Center recognizes those with diabetes who have been insulin-dependent for 25, 50, 75, or 80 years. A: 50-year medal—front. B: 50-year medal—back.

Source: Joslin Diabetes Center.

It Merely Is

"I don't like to think of diabetes as good or bad, it merely is—and produces certain results. If I hadn't had diabetes, I would have been drafted and may not have survived the Vietnam War. My life would have been different in so many ways and looking back to analyze alternatives is pointless. I am very happy where I am and to the extent diabetes was part of getting me here, it has been good."

—Adam Cochran

Menopause

Not only do young women with type 1 diabetes tend to start having their periods later than those without the disease, but they also may go into menopause earlier in life, leading to an overall reduction in the total number of fertile, potentially childbearing years. The reasons for early menopause in type 1 diabetes aren't well understood, though scientists have an idea that it could be related to hormones, autoimmunity, genes, or some combination of factors.

On top of reproductive issues, earlier menopause may have additional health ramifications. Type 1 diabetes already takes a toll on heart health, and early menopause may exacerbate the damage. In women without diabetes, menopause is associated with an increased risk of cardiovascular disease, plus osteoporosis and premature death. Studies haven't actually been done in the context of type 1 diabetes, but it is important to focus on measures to reduce the risk of cardiovascular disease and osteoporosis in post-menopausal woman with type 1 diabetes.

Living Well and Long

The goal for most people as they age is maintaining their independence. On top of all the standard life chores of cooking, shopping, and cleaning, you have the additional jobs of counting carbs, checking blood glucose, and taking insulin. On the other hand, by now these diabetes-related tasks may be second nature to you. With the kids grown up and out of the house, you may have more time for self-care and activities such as yoga, meditation, swimming, or walking with peers. We know the benefits of appropriate exercise and engaging the mind in challenging activities. Who knows, maybe calculating insulin doses helps keep the mind young and functional.

> Working on maintaining core strength and balance is important as people age. Appropriate exercise can help in many ways.

Balance and Exercise

Avoiding falls is a top priority for older adults. A fall can set in motion a series of events that can lead to reduced mobility and a loss of functional independence. Hypoglycemia can trigger a loss of balance and lead to a fall, so check blood glucose regularly. Consume rapid-acting carbohydrates if your blood glucose dips below 70 mg/dL.

Certain medications, such as those taken for high blood pressure, may cause you to become dizzy when standing (postural hypotension), another fall factor. Flexing each ankle 10 times before standing can help prevent this.

Other issues that can impact fall risk include peripheral neuropathy—loss of sensation in the feet and/or a loss of balance (known as proprioception). A reduction in vision can lead to unsteadiness. People with type 1 diabetes seem to develop large-joint issues, and this can lead to pain and disability. A fall and fracture due to osteoporosis can lead to a period of forced immobility, which can be difficult to recover from. Your health-care providers should assess you for these issues.

Keep active, at whatever level is appropriate for you. Sometimes this can be done on your own; other times it requires a caregiver or physical therapist. There are wonderful groups for older folks where physical activity is supervised and is age-appropriate. Pool aerobics can be helpful if walking is difficult due to joint pain or neuropathy. Gentle yoga or Pilates can help with core strengthening. Formal classes exist for balance training as well. Physical therapists can often make house calls and perform physical therapy at your home. Finally, if you have had a heart attack, cardiac rehab is very helpful and a good way to learn healthy exercise habits in a monitored setting.

Not only can physical activity help you maintain balance, it may help slow some of the cognitive decline seen with aging. Walking may be the best, and simplest, exercise for maintaining function, but it's also important to do weight-bearing exercises, such as yoga or using free weights or machines, to maintain bone density and muscle volume. Whatever workout works for you, make sure to start slowly if you're trying something new. Exercise should be challenging, but not too strenuous. Check out NIHseniorHealth.gov and search "exercise."

Nutrition

In our later years, we tend to lose a bit of weight. You may have tooth loss or other dental issues, or trouble with grocery shopping or cooking. Loss of taste and depression may lead you to eat less. Weigh yourself once a week and report any trends of gain or loss to your health-care provider.

Meet with a diabetes nutrition expert to learn how to adjust your meal plan, if needed, as you age. Cognitive impairment can make it more difficult to match carbs to insulin doses, leading to fluctuating blood glucose levels. Eating a diet with consistent carbohydrates can simplify insulin regimens, reducing the possibility of error. If you're not sure how much food you're going to eat at a given meal, it may be wise to take rapid-acting insulin immediately after eating, rather than before. That way you can take a lower dose if you eat less than you'd planned, lowering the risk of hypoglycemia.

Fortified foods and nutritional supplements are another option to meet nutritional needs.

Digging Deep

"It may have been years before I really dug deep into the impact that discovering my condition had on me. Thanks to the unyielding support of my family, I've made it to this point, with 40 years of type 1 under my belt (no pun intended), and a bright future ahead with the help of my pump and continuous glucose monitoring system, and of course, a good attitude and above average cooking skills, if I do say so myself!"

—R. Steven Lewis, 61, is an architect and community planner.

As people with type 1 diabetes get older, rates of low blood surgar reactions increase.

Hypoglycemia

As people with type 1 diabetes age, rates of hypoglycemia increase. Simply increasing the A1C level won't help this problem—people with high A1C values still have low blood glucose levels sometimes. Here are some tips to help make this situation better:

- Eat meals regularly, even if you don't feel hungry. If you don't feel like cooking, there are meals-on-wheels and all sorts of food delivery services that can make eating well easier.
- If your vision is in any way impaired, talk to your diabetes educator or pharmacist about tools you can use to see the numbers on your meter, pens, syringes, and pump. You may need a magnifier or a talking meter.
- If on injections, put different types of insulin in different places in your refrigerator so that they don't get confused. Even young people sometimes get mixed up. It is easy to do and can lead to serious problems if you take too much of the wrong type of insulin.
- Use pen caps that tell you how long it has been since your last dose, to help you remember.
- Talk with your health-care provider about the medications you are taking and whether or not they are interfering with your sensing of low blood glucose levels. There is a class of medication known as β-blockers that can reduce your ability to feel the warning symptoms of a low blood glucose reaction. If you are taking one of these medicines, ask your doctor if there is a substitute. But do NOT stop it on your own, since this could be harmful to your health.

"Helen" is in her 80s. Her A1C is near 6% and she only rarely has low blood glucose reactions. "Beth" is also in her 80s and has dementia and heart disease. She has had frequent, severe low blood glucose reactions that have caused her to fall into a coma. Her doctor has set no A1C target. The goal is to avoid severe lows or dangerous highs. Safety is key in this specific age group.

Solved!

"One of the good things about diabetes is that if you take care of it, you feel better. The results are almost immediate. With a high BG level I feel lousy, irritable, and lethargic. In an hour or two, after taking the appropriate amount of insulin, I'm feeling good again. When I have a low BG, I'm unable to think and am weak and tired. Take some sugar or juice and within ten minutes I'm up and running again. Not many problems in this world are solved so easily or quickly!"

—Sean McLin

Site issues—areas under the skin that are scarred and lumpy—can become limiting issues as people with type 1 diabetes age.

Site Issues

Many older patients have difficulty with their "sites"—the tissues where shots are given and pump catheters are inserted can become spongy and lumpy. This is due to lipohypertrophy, which means that years of putting the insulin (which is a growth factor) under the skin causes the fat cells to grow and expand. The best way to avoid this is to rotate sites frequently, but after many years it may be hard to find an area in which to insert a pump catheter. Hopefully younger generations who have used more pure insulins will have less of a problem with this, but it is important that your health-care provider checks out all of the "pieces" involved in diabetes care, including your fingertips and anywhere you inject insulin or insert a catheter.

Injections and Assisted Living Facilities

Due to the graying of our population, there are now many facilities that cater to the needs of older individuals. These can be assisted living, stepped-care facilities, or board-and-care homes. If you are considering one of these places, carefully research whether or not injections can be given by the level of available staffing. Some of these are not able to accept patients who need help with injectable therapies. If you are helping care for an older loved one with type 1 diabetes, review the diabetes care program that has been followed and help interface between the medical professionals and staff at the facility.

In our experience, we have found the transition to a new residence difficult. But once a new pattern of meals and insulin injections has been established, it often becomes easier, because meals are generally more predictable and staff is available to help.

It is imperative that appropriate use of insulin and timing of SMBG has been arranged with the staff so that no confusion exists. For example, staff needs to understand that long-acting insulin should not be held if a bedtime blood glucose level is considered "too low," because holding long-acting insulin can lead to very high blood glucose levels in the morning.

Nope, Not an iPhone

"I use an insulin pump system that requires a pod placed somewhere on my body, and a PDM on my belt to deliver boluses and monitor the basal delivery. I usually wear the pod on my stomach or on my arm—out of sight to avoid jokes about why I have a computer mouse attached to my body.

I am a docent at an historic house, and tours are supposed to be limited to one hour, which is difficult to do when answering just one question can cause a significant delay. One day a guest with a commitment after the tour just assumed he could do both the tour and keep his commitment. When it became obvious he couldn't, he became agitated and said, 'I have to leave! But I don't want to!' Then he lunged for the PDM on my belt, thinking it was a phone. 'Give me your phone—I'll just inform them I'll be late!' Before I could stop him, my PDM was in his hand and out of its case. He stared at it, flummoxed, and then asked, 'Wow! This must be the new iPhone! How does it work?'"

—Dorena Knepper has had type 1 diabetes since 1984. She worked as an administrator at California State University, Northridge, for over 30 years. She took early retirement in 2005 to indulge her passion for plants and now volunteers in the Children's Garden at the Huntington Library.

Medicare

As anyone who has turned 65 knows, becoming a Medicare recipient is a blessing and a curse. Medicare has very specific rules as to how many blood glucose testing strips people can have per day and whether they will cover an insulin pump or CGM. Fortunately, in response to input from the diabetes community, Medicare is becoming increasingly open to covering technology for seniors. However, there is often more paperwork involved, some of which takes extra time and effort. For instance, nearly all patients with type 1 diabetes need to check their blood glucose levels more than three times per day (the current testing frequency Medicare covers), which means prior authorizations are needed for patients to get more strips. And this isn't something done once, it has to be renewed over and over again, every 3–6 months, for strip and pump coverage. A few companies are now helping people with diabetes to get all of their prescriptions and required diabetes supplies on a routine schedule and ordering their medicines and supplies automatically and notifying them of their availability. Additionally, newer insulins and technologies are very expensive, and older patients living on fixed incomes can have difficulty affording these advances that support improved health and independence.

Eight Hours on the Road

"My wife Judy and I now live in the small town of Lone Pine, California, with our three dogs, eight hens, and an accidental rooster. The population is around 2,000. For me and many rural residents, our primary care is from nurse practitioners, RNs, and physician's assistants.

Both federal and state legislation and policy are written as if everyone has convenient access to services. Medicare requires me to see a diabetes specialist every 3 months to qualify for my insulin pump supplies. That means a 400-mile round-trip drive and 8 hours on the road, not a 20-minute drive across town. I can upload all of the information on my insulin pump to the web in minutes and then send it to my endocrinologist, but no one gets paid to look at it or respond to it. So I drive 200 miles, my pump is uploaded in the office just like I could do at home, and we discuss the results just like we could do online.

Of course there is an advantage to being physically seen by your physician, but before Medicare, I was seeing my doctor only every 6 months. I was able to use a continuous glucose monitor, which Medicare doesn't cover, as well as a pump. I'm grateful for Medicare, but it is a huge bureaucracy with all of the attendant problems."

—Drew Wickman

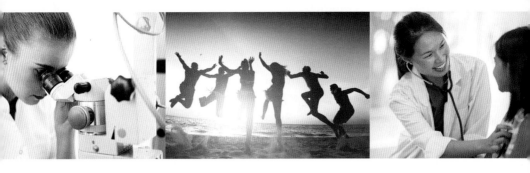

CHAPTER 15

Toward a Cure

You've probably heard this before: The cure for type 1 diabetes is just 10 years away! We're not going to set up any false expectations in this chapter. However, all over the world, researchers are searching for a cure and treatments to prevent type 1 diabetes, and ways to improve health and quality of life of people with diabetes. Some of this science looks promising.

Getting a new technology from the laboratory to a patient is an extremely long and difficult process, both scientifically and with respect to regulation. A new treatment must prove itself to be safe and effective. Another potential roadblock, since so many cases of type 1 diabetes start during childhood, is that studies may need to be done in children as well as adults.

> There are hundreds of ways to cure type 1 diabetes in a rodent, but none in a human.

If you want to know how to interpret "breakthroughs" that are constantly reported in the media, first look at the species in which the "miracle cure" occurs. There are hundreds of ways in which to cure type 1 diabetes in rodents, but they have different immune systems than humans. However, rodents are generally the first mammals studied. The next tests tend to be done in rabbits, which is a step closer. Then in dogs, pigs, primates, and finally humans. Testing doesn't always go in this sequence, and steps are often omitted, but try not to get overly excited until a new approach is tested in phase 1 studies in actual humans. That tells you there is a chance. In phase 1, the new drug is tested in people who don't have diabetes to be sure it isn't toxic—this is a step purely for safety and is done in maybe 30–80 people.

If the drug doesn't seem to have any immediate safety concerns, it moves to phase 2 studies, which involve maybe 300 people who have type 1 diabetes. Phase 2 is a start to look at whether the drug works—is it effective against the disease?

179

Finally, phase 3 studies, which may be in a few thousand people, improve the knowledge of both safety and effectiveness of the treatment. Finally, after all of these steps, the data is submitted to the Food and Drug Administration (FDA), and the drug is either approved, sent back for more studies, or rejected. These steps take many years. Most experimental drugs never make it to phase 1 trials. If you want to know what new treatment is close to being available, check out the drugs in phase 2 or phase 3 studies. The NIH lists all of the research trials that are going on in the United States and can be searched at ClinicalTrials.gov. Participating in a research study is often a good way to help in the development of new treatments. The steps for approving devices, like pumps and sensors, is different than that for medications, but all of it takes testing, time, and patience.

"Artificial Pancreas"

It's a bit of a stretch to call the artificial pancreas **(Fig. 15.1)**, more recently renamed "automated insulin delivery system," a cure. But for those who have tested them, these devices can be a game changer, particularly in the right setting. In the future, artificial pancreases may be more like what you might imagine: implantable synthetic organs that make diabetes disappear. However, the versions in development today are not so dissimilar from products you're already familiar with: an insulin pump and a continuous glucose monitor. The magic difference is an algorithm—a computer program—that takes the readings from CGM, does a little math, and then tells the pump how much insulin to deliver.

The first FDA-approved iteration of a system that provides automated insulin delivery is called a hybrid closed-loop system (HCL). A "full-on" system would administer insulin (and glucagon) throughout the day and night, controlling all

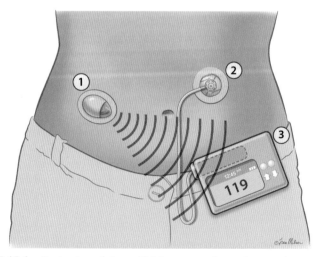

FIGURE 15.1   Illustration of the artificial pancreas. 1. continuous glucose sensor, 2. infusion set, 3. insulin pump.

the basal and bolus insulin dosing automatically, without a required input for mealtime dosing. Such a system has been developed and is being tested and refined. The HCL system consists of an insulin pump, sensor, and control algorithm that raises and lowers the basal rate in response to changes in blood glucose levels. The user still must carb count and enter bolus doses, but the system takes care of the rest. It is particularly helpful in stabilizing overnight blood glucose levels and helps catch rising or falling blood glucose levels between meals. More types of HCL systems are being developed and studied, and each new generation should be better than the last.

> The available "artificial pancreas" system still requires that the user enter their carbohydrates and calibrate the sensor, but for the right person it can make life with diabetes better.

The problem with all of these systems is that they depend on the devices working—that there are no clogs in the insulin infusion set, that the sensor is accurately reading your glucose level, that you are making sure the "pieces" of the system are working and talking to each other. It also means that there are no infusion site or tape issues and each part of the system can be kept fully functional. Therefore, both people with diabetes and their providers will need to be fully educated on how to use these systems and be ready to troubleshoot if difficulties arise. The decision to use such a system should be made individually—for some, particularly adults on a stable basal insulin, overnight variability is not much of a problem and blood glucose goals can be reached and maintained with a multiple injection regimen and a CGM; for others this technology will be a welcome addition to stabilizing overnight glucose levels and aiding in their diabetes management. Regardless of individual preference, however, the approval of the first HCL system is a big step forward in the development and use of diabetes technology.

Five Days of Freedom

"My daughter Adalyne, then 11, got the opportunity to wear a dual-hormone bionic pancreas (now called iLet) as part of a summer camp study. It was an experience of a lifetime.

The belt around her waist held two insulin pumps— one for insulin and one for glucagon—a CGM receiver, and a cell phone. It looked heavy and bulky, but she didn't seem to mind. It also required daily glucagon site changes and patience, as the equipment required being attached to a wall connector for charging.

For five days, Adalyne was granted freedom from the mental burden of constantly thinking about her glucose levels. She ate without counting carbohydrates, slept without worrying about what would happen to her blood sugar overnight, and participated in camp activities without feeling limited by her numbers.

When I arrived to pick her up, she couldn't wait to show me the system and excitedly began telling me stories. I watched in awe as she ate lunch without counting carbs for the first time in nearly a decade, then tried not to panic when she didn't finish everything on her plate in favor of hugging her cabin-mates goodbye. After lunch, we wandered outside and she started playing a game with the other study participants. It was the first time in her entire life that I watched her play without thinking about how her blood sugars were doing. I was captivated by her ability to run, jump, and play ball with her friends. I watched the concentration on her face instead of trying to interpret her expression as a nonverbal cue of hypoglycemia. I noticed her strong muscles and marveled at her flexibility without wondering if I should have decreased the basal rate on her insulin pump. I laughed at her natural clumsiness instead of rushing to her side with a juice box thinking it was a symptom of low blood sugar. For the first time since her diagnosis, I had no idea what her blood sugar was or how it had been trending, and it felt like freedom.

I felt a heaviness in my gut as the clock ticked closer to 3 p.m. I knew each second was creeping closer to the moment we would have to return the device. When the time came, my daughter scooted next to me and reluctantly began removing each part. One by one, she handed everything back. My heart broke when her tears came. She felt it too ... the 'normalcy,' the freedom, the hope. We put her usual Animas pump back on, and bid farewell to camp—both of us forever changed by the experience, and excited about the future.”

—Wendy Rose, a registered nurse since 1995,
says that nothing in nursing school prepared her for
Adalyne's diagnosis at age 2.

Smart Insulin

Researchers are working on a “smart” insulin that would be injected, keep circulating in the body, and be activated as needed when blood glucose levels rise, and switch off again when blood glucose levels return to normal. A smart insulin would eliminate extreme high and low blood glucose levels. This work is looking at a single injection per day or even one injection per week.

β-CELL REPLACEMENT

Type 1 diabetes is an autoimmune disease that attacks the insulin-producing β-cells in the pancreas, rendering them incapable of keeping up with the demands of the body. So one way to cure diabetes would be to replace the lost β-cells and keep the replacements from getting destroyed anew by the immune system. Researchers are working on a number of strategies to replace β-cells in people with type 1 diabetes, but at least one strategy has been around since the 1970s: pancreas transplant.

Pancreas Transplants

An organ transplant is a big deal. Not only is it major surgery—with the inherent surgery-related risks—but organ recipients must take medications that suppress their immune systems for the rest of their lives. That being said, for the right patient, pancreas transplants are the most effective means we have for restoring insulin production in the body. People who've had successful pancreas transplants can stop taking insulin, measuring blood glucose levels, and living like they have type 1 diabetes. A pancreas transplant takes care of all that, liberating recipients from the disease. However, not all pancreas transplants take, and some fail over time.

There are three types of pancreas transplants:

- Simultaneous pancreas and kidney transplant (SPK)
- Pancreas after kidney transplant (PAK)
- Pancreas transplant alone (PTA)

SPKs have the greatest success rates, with 72% still operational at 5 years. PAKs failure rates are a little higher than SPKs, and PTAs have the highest failure rates of all, with only half of the transplants surviving for five years. The procedures have varying failure rates due to differences in how the immune system responds to each type of transplant, as well as to details related to the surgical procedures themselves.

Not everyone with type 1 diabetes is a candidate for a pancreas transplant, and they are typically reserved for those with blood glucose levels that are erratic and very difficult to manage. Because simultaneous pancreas and kidney transplants have the highest success rates, the ideal candidate for a pancreas transplant would be someone with kidney failure. Another advantage of SPK is that a person who needs kidney transplant already faces the risks of surgery and lifelong immune suppressive therapy, so the pancreas can come along for free. Candidates must also have excellent cardiovascular health, which may be an issue for people with type 1 diabetes. A third issue is supply: there are only ~1,400 potentially suitable donor pancreases available in the U.S. each year. On the bright side, insurance will typically cover pancreas transplants for suitable candidates.

Do-It-Yourself "Artificial Pancreas"

"I am one of the lucky ones. I have access to insulin, an insulin pump, and a continuous glucose monitor. However, I still worried that it wasn't enough. A CGM is only as good as your ability to hear the alarms to know that you need to take action. And I sleep through CGM alarms. Deep inside, I worried about what would happen if I had a bad low and did not wake up, especially because I was living by myself.

I talked to CGM manufacturers and asked them to make louder alarms. I was given a range of responses, from 'It's loud enough' to explanations about alarm volume being a trade-off against battery life.

One day, I saw someone on Twitter share a post about pulling his son's CGM data and sending it to the cloud. That same day, I reached out to him and asked him to share his computer code so my computer could do the same thing.

I was able to send my CGM data to an app on my phone to make louder alarms that I didn't sleep through, and create a webpage to share my data with my loved ones. To prevent them from getting every alarm, I added buttons to the page to "snooze" the alarms based on the actions I took. Along with Scott Leibrand, I then built an algorithm using information about my actions (insulin taken and/or food eaten), and sent additional alarms suggesting further action only when needed.

I then decided to use other tools shared openly online to help my CGM communicate directly with my pump. With some additional hardware, we 'closed the loop' and automatically sent temporary basal rates to my pump to increase or decrease the insulin I was getting, based on the changes in my blood glucose. It has been amazing to have a system that automatically keeps my blood glucose in range.

With access to my data, I went from building a louder alarm system that could wake me up to building an automated insulin delivery system that allows me to safely sleep at night! And in the spirit of open source, which enabled me to build these systems, we called this OpenAPS, or an open-source artificial pancreas system, and have published a reference design, code, and documentation for anyone who also wants to build their own system before a commercially approved system becomes available."

—@DanaMLewis is a creator and founder of the
#OpenAPS movement.

Islet Transplants

To bypass the need for major surgery, researchers have been developing ways to transplant only the islets, without the rest of the pancreas. Islets are the clusters of cells in the pancreas that house the β-cells. Islet transplantation goes a little something like this: The first step is to extract the islets from a donor pancreas, being careful to collect as many as possible without damaging the delicate clusters. With islet transplantation, numbers matter. A healthy, normal-size pancreas holds ~1 million islets. A 150-pound person needs ~600,000–700,000 donor islets to normalize blood glucose levels. These cells are introduced directly into the portal vein, a main blood vessel in the liver. The islets then implant themselves inside the liver's tiny blood vessels, where they begin to make insulin in response to high blood glucose levels.

Just as with pancreas transplants, people with islet transplants need to take immunosuppressive drugs to reduce the immune response that would kill off the donated islet cells. These drugs have many side effects. Therefore, deciding whether it is better to have type 1 diabetes or take strong drugs that suppress the immune system is not simple.

The life span of these cells under current transplant protocols falls far short of that achieved with whole-organ transplants, but improvements are coming. The most promising results to date showed that, after three years, ~45% of people who received islet transplants still maintained normal blood glucose levels without taking insulin (but taking immunosuppressive drugs).

Islet transplantation remains an experimental procedure and so is rarely covered by insurance. That may change in the coming years, as the FDA evaluates results from an ongoing multicenter trial aimed at standardizing islet transplant procedures. However, islet transplantation suffers the same drawback as organ transplantation: a limited supply of donor pancreases.

Shining Moment

"After completing a series of questionnaires and interviews and undergoing a variety of tests, I was accepted to the transplant program being conducted at various medical centers by the Clinical Islet Transplantation Consortium. After waiting for 2.5 years, I received a call in March 2010 that a donor pancreas was available. I took a train from D.C. to the University of Pennsylvania in Philadelphia and spent a couple of days in the hospital being prepared for the transplant. My immune system was suppressed with powerful drugs, and a surgeon injected the cells into my liver through a tiny incision. I remained in the hospital for a number of days following the transplant.

I continued to take insulin for approximately 6 weeks after the transplant to provide the islets time to become adjusted to their new home. Luckily, the islet cells appeared to thrive, and insulin was now being produced. My blood sugars were almost always in a nondiabetic range. But for the islets to function, I had to take immunosuppressant drugs to ensure that my own system would not reject them. As a consequence, I did have a variety of adverse effects, including tremors, cold sores, and periodic dizziness when I stood up too suddenly. But these were all small prices to pay for what seemed to be a different life—a life that I never thought possible.

In the autumn of 2011, I began to feel a bit under the weather. I found that it was becoming more difficult to get up and down stairs without losing my breath. Eventually, I asked my family to call an ambulance.

Over the next couple weeks, I visited emergency rooms at two other hospitals. Though doctors knew of my immunocompromised state, I was diagnosed with a form of community pneumonia and was given various antibiotics. I failed to get better. I was finally transported by ambulance from D.C. to the Hospital of the University of Pennsylvania. As I was being loaded into the ambulance, a doctor told my wife that a helicopter should have been sent because he wasn't sure I would make it to the Penn Hospital alive.

I spent 10 days in Penn's hospital and was often in a semiconscious state. Halfway through my time there, I was finally diagnosed with pneumocystis pneumonia, a diagnosis that is often associated with those whose immune systems are compromised, such as HIV and AIDs patients. I believe the medical community failed me by not quickly associating my compromised immune system with the possibility of having PCP. The drugs used to treat community pneumonia do not adequately treat PCP. As a result, I came pretty close to dying.

I recovered after receiving the proper diagnosis and the correct antibiotic. My islets remained active for another 6 months or so. But eventually they died, and my brief shining moment on the hill ended. So I am back to my pumping, fingerpricking, carbcounting type 1 life. I am grateful for my existence, but I still hope for the cure."

—Andy Gordon, 62, is a librarian and volunteers at the Smithsonian.

Making β-Cells

Pig islets are being studied as potential replacements for human islets, but there are drawbacks of using tissues from other species, such as the potential for cross-species disease transmission.

Another approach is to make islets in the laboratory. Embryonic stem cells are special cells that have the malleability to turn into any of the body's cell types if given the right conditions under which to grow. Scientists across the globe are tinkering with stem cells, delivering various nutrients, enzymes, and other factors at precise times over the course of the cells' maturation to produce a healthy culture of the desired cell types.

Several teams have successfully turned stem cells into insulin-producing β-cells in the laboratory. They've even reversed diabetes in mice, though these mice had poorly developed immune systems. This brings us back to the same problem that pancreas and islet transplants face: the immune system.

Once you get insulin-producing cells into the body, how do you protect them from the immune system? There are immune-suppressing medications, which aren't ideal because they have side effects and have a tendency to fail. An alternative approach is encapsulation. Imagine a tiny pouch with pores big enough to let glucose in and insulin out, but small enough to keep β-cells in while keeping killer immune system cells out.

STOPPING THE IMMUNE ATTACK

β-Cell preservation, rather than replacement, is yet another path to a cure, and may also help prevent type 1 in those at risk of the disease. In theory, stopping the autoimmune process that destroys β-cells in its tracks should *1)* prevent the ongoing annihilation of insulin-producing cells and *2)* allow those cells to regenerate.

Scientists have studied different agents to protect β-cells in people with type 1 diabetes. The studies have had varying success, and none have demonstrated the sort of lasting benefits that could be considered a cure. At best, some approaches seem to extend the lives of β-cells, maintaining residual insulin production for longer than placebo. While not a cure, even these small successes may improve lives.

But turning those small successes into a cure is going to be a long road. Just designing a study that can assess a particular therapy is fraught with challenges. Dose, delivery strategy (oral vs. injection, etc.), target population (adult vs. child, early-onset vs. long-duration, etc.), and timing of treatments can all have an effect on the outcome of a study—get one variable wrong, and a promising therapy may not work, or may not work up to its potential.

The treatment approaches that are under investigation are based, in part, on our understanding of how the immune system targets and destroys β-cells in type 1 diabetes. Many of these strategies focus on ways to generally or selectively suppress the β-cell–destroying behavior of the immune system. The gist of this process is that immune system cells called "antigen-presenting cells" begin to recognize pieces of the β-cells as foreign. That's bad news. These antigen-presenting cells then recruit other immune system cells, called T-cells, to find and kill β-cells.

Antigen-Based Therapies

Some of the type 1 treatments under study focus on the antigen side of this problem: Can we get the antigen-presenting cells to accept β-cells as part of the family? An antigen is any biological bit—whether from a cell, bacteria, virus, or whatever—that spurs the immune system into action. Insulin is recognized as an antigen in many people with type 1 diabetes, which is one way the immune system targets the insulin-producing β-cells.

Researchers have attempted to give insulin—orally or nasally—to people at high risk of developing type 1 diabetes and to those with new-onset disease. The hope is that the body could get comfortable with insulin and stop attacking the cells that make it. Scientists are also studying a handful of other type 1 diabetes antigens. In addition, some emerging research suggests that agents that decommission the antigen-presenting cells themselves could prevent or treat type 1 diabetes.

Targeting T-Cells

Treatments that target the T-cells involve immunosuppression. General immunosuppressants, such as cyclosporine, can knock out T-cells, as well as the rest of the immune system. Some experimental drugs—targeted immunosuppressants—use a bit more finesse. They attempt to block communication between T-cells and antigen-presenting cells so the T-cells don't get the message that they are supposed to kill β-cells. These signal blockers are lab-generated antibodies, special proteins that recognize and stick to specific pieces of the T-cell, shutting down their tendency to kill β-cells.

Another T-cell–based strategy targets yet another immune system cell, called a T regulatory cell (Treg). Like the name suggests, Tregs are like shepherds to the T-cell herd. In mouse studies, bumping up the population of Tregs reversed type 1 diabetes. Early human trials that deliver Tregs directly or involve agents that promote growth of native Treg populations are currently underway.

Inflammation

The process that vanquishes β-cells includes an inflammation component, leading scientists to look at anti-inflammatory agents as possible treatments for type 1.

PREVENTION

Both genetic and environmental factors play a role in type 1 diabetes. Since we can't do anything about our genes, researchers are trying to identify the environmental factors that contribute to type 1 diabetes, and to snuff them out in those at high risk of developing the disease. A smattering of studies are looking at dietary factors—could eating a certain way in early life help prevent type 1 diabetes?

Dairy

Breast-feeding is linked to a lower risk of developing type 1 diabetes, but it's still unclear why. Some evidence suggests that introducing cow's milk, and specifically cow proteins, into a baby's diet at an early age may confuse the immune system, leading to type 1 diabetes later in life. To test this hypothesis, the Trial to Reduce Insulin-Dependent Diabetes Mellitus in the Genetically at Risk is comparing the risk of type 1 diabetes in babies fed cow's milk formula and those given a "highly hydrolyzed" formula that doesn't contain intact cow proteins. Final results are expected in 2017.

Good Fats

Another study is checking whether a diet high in omega-3 fatty acids, such as docoshexaenoic acid (DHA), can lower the risk of type 1. In the study, infants received DHA supplements until 36 months of age. The researchers are watching these children as they grow up to see if they are protected from type 1.

LOOK TO THE FUTURE, LIVE IN THE PRESENT

Researchers are working on better ways to treat and cure type 1 diabetes. Progress has been made in both areas, although improvements in treatment are advancing more rapidly than finding a cure. The cure, as discussed previously, will likely come from the field of immunology—finding a way to selectively change the immune system so that the body doesn't destroy its own β-cells. The people who figure this out will have the key to dealing with many different diseases. In addition to curing diabetes, figuring out how to selectively turn off parts of the immune system might cure celiac and Hashimoto's disease, lupus, multiple sclerosis, and rheumatoid arthritis, among others.

But the immune system is tough to manipulate. For now, treatments ranging from better insulins to more sophisticated delivery devices to possible β-cell replacement are closer to being available.

Although managing diabetes is a constant challenge, diabetes is a treatable disease, even if not curable. Living life with type 1 diabetes *is* getting easier—think about how much has changed in the past decade. People can live full, long, healthy lives with type 1 diabetes. They don't have to feel limited as to what they can do in their lives. The future is bright.

In the end, the best approach is to hope for a cure but live in the moment. As you face the challenges of living with type 1 diabetes, realize that there are many of us in the diabetes community who are cheering you on.

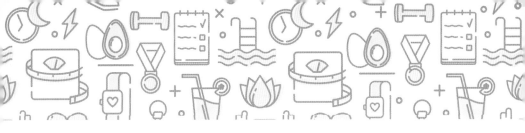

Appendix

Sources for Type 1 Diabetes Information

Diabetes.org	American Diabetes Association's mission is to prevent and cure diabetes and to improve the lives of all people affected by this disease.
JDRF.org	JDRF's mission is to accelerate life-changing breakthroughs to cure, prevent, and treat type 1 diabetes and its complications.
MyGlu.org	Glu is an on-line community designed to accelerate research and amplify voices of those living with type 1 diabetes
DiabetesEducator.org	American Association of Diabetes Educators. Resources for patients, including "Find a Diabetes Educator."
EatRight.org	Academy of Nutrition and Dietetics. Click on "Find an Expert," enter your zip and refine your search by specialty.
NIHseniorHealth.gov	National Institutes of Health, Senior Health. Information for older adults from the National Institutes of Health.
NIDDK.nih.gov	National Institute of Diabetes and Digestive and Kidney Diseases.
ClinicalTrials.gov	Registry and results database of publicly and privately supported clinical studies of human participants conducted around the world.

Popular Type 1 Diabetes Magazines and Blogs

This is not an inclusive list. Many of these have associated Twitter feeds, Instagrams, etc.

ASweetLife.org	DiabetesSportsProject.com
BetaCellPodcast.com	diaTribe.org
BeyondType1.org	dLife.com
ChildrenWithDiabetes.com	Healthline.com/diabetesmine
CollegeDiabetesNetwork.org	InsulinNation.com
DiabetesSisters.org	Taking Control of Your Diabetes: TCOYD.org

Personal Type 1 Diabetes Blogs

Too numerous to list. There are hundreds of people with type 1 diabetes who share their experiences with great wit, insight, and sincerity. We recommend that you search for and read the blogs that speak to you personally. Please note that most of these bloggers are not health care professionals and are sharing their own personal experiences. It is wise to talk with your diabetes team before following any recommendations in a blog.

Consortia Studying Type 1 Diabetes

TEDDY	The Environmental Determinants of Diabetes in the Young	The primary objective(s) of TEDDY is the identification of infectious agents, dietary factors, or other environmental exposures that are associated with increased risk of autoimmunity and T1D.	teddy.epi.usf.edu
nPOD	Network for Pancreatic Organ Donors with Diabetes	The mission of nPOD is to characterize pancreata and related tissues from organ donors with T1D or who are islet autoantibody positive and utilize the tissues to address key immunological, histological, viral, and metabolic questions related to how type 1 diabetes develops.	jdrfnPOD.org
SEARCH	SEARCH for Diabetes in Youth	SEARCH is a national, multicenter study aimed at understanding more about diabetes among children and young adults in the United States.	SearchForDiabetes.org
TrialNet	Type 1 Diabetes TrialNet	TrialNet is an international network of researchers who are exploring ways to prevent, delay, and reverse the progression of type 1 diabetes.	DiabetesTrialNet.org

(Continiued)

Consortia Studying Type 1 Diabetes (Cont.)

ITN	Immune Tolerance Network	The purpose of ITN is to understand and achieve immune tolerance to prevent and cure human disease.	ImmuneTolerance.org
TRIGR	Trial to Reduce IDDM in the Genetically at Risk	TRIGR tested whether weaning to a casein hydrolysate formula during the first 6–8 months of life—in place of cow's milk–based formula—reduced the incidence of autoimmunity and type 1 diabetes in genetically susceptible newborn infants. Results expected in 2017.	trigr.epi.usf.edu
DirecNet	Diabetes Research in Children Network	This research study examines differences in brain structure and brain function in young children with type 1 diabetes as compared with non-diabetic controls over time.	DirecNet.stanford.edu
T1D Exchange	T1D Exchange	Clinic registry bolsters research and development projects and programs in type 1 diabetes by helping researchers characterize individuals living with the disease, conduct exploratory or hypothesis-generating analyses, and identify participants for future clinical studies.	T1Dexchange.org

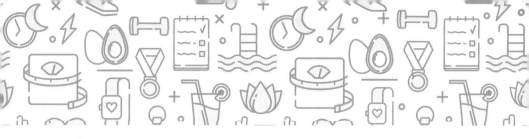

Index